CR ConsumerReports™

SHOULD I EAT THIS?

Simple ways to know what to eat and what to avoid.

From the Editors of Consumer Reports On Health

Consumer Reports *Should I Eat This?* is published by Consumer
Reports, Inc., a nonprofit, independent organization that was
established in 1936 to provide consumers with information and
advice on products, services, health, and personal finance.

The information contained in this book is not intended to
substitute for professional or medical advice. Consumer
Reports disclaims responsibility or liability for any loss that
may be incurred as a result of the use or application of any
information included in Consumer Reports *Should I Eat This?*
Readers should always consult their physicians or other
professionals for treatment and advice.

SHOULD I EAT THIS?

INTRODUCTION

If you have ever paused before biting into a food and wondered, *Should I Eat This?* — then this book if for you.

It has the answer to that question, plus many other questions about what you *should* eat and *should not* eat.

Are there really foods that keep you young? Is a cup of coffee good for you, or bad? What about a glass of wine? What's the healthiest breakfast cereal? How can you tell if the beef you are eating is safe and free of harmful antibiotics? What's the truth about gluten? Omega-3s? Green tea?

Consumer Reports' team of M.Ds, Ph.Ds, nutritionists, editors, and taste-testers analyze the research, cut through the jargon, and separate food facts from fiction. You get clear advice, recommendations, and the answer to the question *Should I Eat This?*

The facts you learn from *Should I Eat This?* can have an enormous impact on both your long- and short-term health. You'll find a dietary approach to help reduce the risk of serious disease and the unwanted effects of aging. Even everyday ailments may resolve themselves with simple dietary adjustments.

One thing we never lose sight of is the enjoyment that food can and should provide. That's why we reveal which foods rated highest in our blind taste tests for both taste and nutrition. And we provide recipes with ingredients you should eat, not just for your good health, but because they taste great too.

CHAPTER ONE

START

Eat *THIS*
to lower your blood pressure

Eating 1½ apples a day *does* keep the doctor away: Researchers found that people who get 1½ servings of fruit a day reduce their risk of fatal heart disease by 27 percent and stroke by 40 percent compared to people who never eat fruit. One possible reason: Fruit eaters had significantly lower blood pressure.

IN THIS CHAPTER:

EAT *FOOD*, NOT SUPPLEMENTS

Getting the right nutrients, at the right time in your life, is one of the major keys to good health. The secret here is to get them from food, not supplements.

Research has found that eating whole foods provides a wide range of health benefits that supplements haven't been able to match.

ONE SUPPLEMENT YOU SHOULD NOT TAKE: VITAMIN E

Vitamin E supplements are said by some to help prevent cancer, dementia, and heart disease, but there's little proof— and plenty of reason to avoid them.

Research has linked regular use to a 13 percent higher risk of heart failure in certain populations. A study published in the *Journal of the American Medical Association (JAMA)* in 2011 also found that taking 400 IU daily may boost the likelihood of prostate cancer by 17 percent. Vitamin E supplements may also make some chemotherapy drugs less effective. Who might need them? Our experts don't recommend them for anyone.

Perhaps it is the full complement of the nutrients in plant foods — working together — that makes eating a wide variety of foods more beneficial than taking supplements of individual nutrients.

WHAT YOU SHOULD KNOW ABOUT SUPPLEMENTS

Vitamins and minerals are marketed as products that help keep you healthy. But some may carry more risks than benefits, especially as we age.

"Supplements are most useful when they're used to replace dietary deficiencies. Therefore, most of us don't need them. Such needless use can be harmful, especially if you also take prescription medications," says Consumer Reports' chief medical adviser, Marvin M. Lipman, M.D.

In addition, the evidence supporting supplements is often flimsy or mixed, and because of lax regulation, you can't always be sure what they contain. The following three supplements, (as well as vitamin E, see page 4), may be especially harmful to your health if you're over 50.

1. Folic Acid (Folate)

It has been suggested — but not proven — that folic acid (vitamin B9) may ward off Alzheimer's disease, depression, and heart disease. But a recent study published by the *American Journal of Clinical Nutrition* links excess folate (including folic acid) to burning, tingling, or numbness in the extremities of people with a common gene variant.

"The odds were sevenfold higher for those who consumed more than 800 mcg daily," says co-author Ligi Paul, Ph.D., of the Jean Mayer USDA Human Nutrition Research Center on Aging at Tufts University.

In addition, taking as little as 300 mcg daily may mask a B12 deficiency, which is relatively common in older adults. If undiagnosed, that can lead to nerve damage, cognitive trouble, and even psychiatric problems. Folic acid can also reduce the effectiveness of the seizure drug fosphenytoin (*Cerebyx*® and generic) and the cancer drug methotrexate (*Rheumatrex*® and generic).

Who might need it? Women who are pregnant or planning to get pregnant, to prevent birth defects.

2. Calcium

You might take calcium supplements to strengthen your bones, which can weaken with age. But regular use may increase the risk of kidney stones and possibly heart disease. A study in the *Journal of the American Heart Association* in October 2016 found that people who took calcium supplements over a 10-year period were more likely to accumulate artery clogging plaque that can lead to heart attacks than those who did not take calcium. Supplemental calcium can also negatively interact with some heart and thyroid medications.

Who might need it? People who eat little or no calcium-rich food, such as dairy products and leafy greens.

3. Iron

Anemia, or low blood levels of iron, is more common with age. But taking too much iron can mask symptoms of anemia, which can be caused by internal bleeding, and lead to a missed diagnosis. Iron supplements can also inhibit the absorption of certain antibiotics and blood pressure-lowering drugs such as captopril (*Capoten®* and generic). And if you have hemochromatosis, a surprisingly common genetic condition that causes the body to deposit excess iron in vital organs, taking iron pills can lead to an overload of the mineral, potentially causing diabetes symptoms, heart problems, and liver damage.

Who might need it? People with diagnosed iron-deficiency anemia.

Manufacturers aren't required to prove that their products are safe or work as advertised before they reach the marketplace.

The Food and Drug Administration (FDA) does not usually test supplements to make sure they contain only the ingredients on the label. That means you can't be exactly sure what you're getting when you take them. Even worse, in some cases manufacturers add illegal or prescription medications to their supplements. In other cases, supplements may contain naturally occurring substances that are chemically identical to pharmaceutical products. And you may not know this.

"Researchers have found prescription medications, banned pharmaceuticals, and drugs that have never been tested in humans in supplements," says dietary supplement safety expert Pieter Cohen, M.D., an assistant professor at Harvard Medical School. Those substances could interact with medications you take, cause negative side effects, or lead to dangerously high doses of medicine.

When asking yourself the question *Should I Eat This?* always start with food, not supplements.

Foods help you reap benefits that you might expect to get from supplements. Take produce for example:

Eating roughly 10 servings of fruits and veggies per day could significantly cut your risk of heart disease, stroke, cancer, and early death according to to an analysis of 95 studies published in 2017 by researchers at Imperial College, London. But even a small amount is far better than none.

Protect your heart: Researchers say that having 2.5 daily servings (a small piece of fruit or ½ cup of cooked veggies is one serving) could reduce heart disease risk by 16 percent and stroke risk by 18 percent.

Strive for variety: Researchers found that apples, pears, citrus, leafy greens, and crucifers such as broccoli and cauliflower reduced the risk of heart disease.

FOR A COLD OR FLU:

Eat THIS
Chicken soup

No food has been proven to shorten the duration of a cold, but research shows that chicken soup really may help ease the sneezing, sore throat, and stuffy nose caused by inflammation. See our Homemade Chicken Soup recipe on page 126.

Skip THIS
Echinacea, ginseng, vitamin C, and zinc

These supplements have often been touted for cold prevention and symptom control. But research results on the effectiveness of all have been mixed.

Save your money. Supplements are not thoroughly regulated by the FDA, and as a result, researchers can't draw firm conclusions from data. Avoid zinc-based nasal sprays altogether. The FDA says that they may permanently destroy your sense of smell.

FOR OSTEOARTHRITIS PAIN:

Eat THIS
Turmeric

Research suggests that curcumin, a substance that gives turmeric its yellow color, may ease osteoarthritis symptoms. Turmeric is a staple in Indian curries and mustard.

Not THIS
Glucosamine, chondroitin, fish oil

Some people use supplements such as glucosamine and chondroitin (often together) or fish oil for joint pain caused by osteoarthritis. But, so far studies have shown that glucosamine and chondroitin are no more effective than a placebo. Plus fish-oil supplements can cause side effects such as diarrhea and stomach pain.

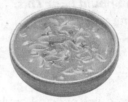

FOR SEXUAL ENHANCEMENT:

Drink *THIS*
Coffee

Caffeine may promote penile blood flow. A study found that men who consume 170 to 375 milligrams of caffeine per day — equivalent to about 2 to 3 cups of coffee — were about 40 percent less likely to have erectile dysfunction than men who took in much less.

Don't take *THESE*
Sex supplements

In a recent study that analyzed 150 dietary supplements marketed to increase sexual performance, all of which claimed to only contain natural ingredients, two-thirds were found to be adulterated with drugs.

Some of the ingredients were unapproved and untested, but prescription erectile dysfunction drugs sildenafil (*Viagra*), tadalafil (*Cialis*), and vardenafil (*Levitra*) were also frequently found.

Supplements that contain prescription ED drugs can cause dizziness, headache, flushing, stomach upset, and blurred vision. They can also lead to dangerously low blood pressure and death when combined with heart medications such as nitrates or nitroglycerin.

FOR HEART HEALTH:

Eat *THIS*
Salmon

Eating two or more servings per week of oily fish is linked with a lower risk of heart attack and stroke. Fish that are rich in omega-3s include wild salmon and sardines. They are both low in mercury, and wild salmon has fewer PCBs than farmed.

Not *THIS*
Fish oil supplements

Our bodies need the omega-3 fatty acids fish-oil pills contain, but most people are better off getting them from fatty fish — not from supplements. The latest evidence suggests that fish-oil pills don't offer the same protection as food, even for people at risk for heart disease.

ARE SUPPLEMENTS EVER A GOOD IDEA?

For now, we recommend skipping supplements unless a doctor says you need them for a specific health condition. Instead, get your vitamins and minerals from a healthy diet, including vegetables, fruits, whole grains, and lean proteins.

So, while most of us get the vitamins and minerals we need from food, you might want to ask your doctor about:

Vitamin D: If you've been diagnosed with osteoporosis, get little sunlight, or rarely consume vitamin D-rich foods such as fatty fish, eggs, and fortified milk.

AREDS2: (a blend of vitamins C and E, copper, lutein, zeaxanthin, and zinc) If you have age-related macular degeneration, a leading cause of vision loss.

Vitamin B12: If you're a strict vegan, or if you regularly take certain kinds of heartburn drugs or metformin, a diabetes medication.

EASY WAYS TO EAT HEALTHY NOW

You don't need to overhaul your diet. These changes deliver big benefits but take very little effort.

Setting a goal of eating better often inspires people to attempt a big change in their habits. But those intentions fail more often than not.

"People set unrealistic goals and attempt to make wholesale changes," says Lesley Lutes, Ph.D., associate professor of psychology at the University of British Columbia. "That all-or-nothing behavior becomes overwhelming, leaves you feeling deprived, and sets you up for failure." That's why we are advocating a more realistic approach using the 4 steps below.

SMART EATING *CAN* BE SIMPLE.

1. *Try making a few minor tweaks first.* That helps the changes feel doable, not daunting, and you will still see improvements in your health. "You have so many diet choices to make every day, so even if you make a change only some of the time, the benefits add up," Lutes says.

A recent study by researchers at the University of South Australia supports that strategy. They found that replacing just 25 percent of discretionary foods (such as dessert, snacks, and sugary beverages) with healthy foods resulted in a huge improvement in overall diet quality — reducing sugars intake by almost 21 percent and calories by almost 4 percent, and increasing protein intake by about 2 percent.

That means that something as simple as trading a few cookies for a piece of fruit, a handful of chips for some fresh veggies, or a soda for a glass of sparkling water, can make a big difference.

2. *Eat More Unprocessed Whole Grains.* You know that whole grains provide you with fiber and other nutrients. To many people, eating more whole grains means eating whole-wheat bread and pasta in place of the regular versions. Though switching from products made with refined white flour to those made with whole-grain flours is a good start, focusing on eating actual whole grains in their natural forms is better for your health.

"They've been tied to so many health benefits, including reducing the risk of cardiovascular disease, stroke, type 2 diabetes, and cancer," says Frank Hu, M.D., Ph.D., a professor of nutrition and epidemiology at the Harvard T.H. Chan School of Public Health.

Brown rice, buckwheat, farro, millet, oats, wheat berries, and other grains are considered "whole" because they contain the entire kernel— the endosperm, bran, and germ — so they provide a variety of phytonutrients and fiber, which may reduce your risk for certain conditions. Amaranth and quinoa count as whole grains, even though they are actually seeds.

All three components of the kernel are also found in some processed whole-grain foods. But the data suggest that we should be eating most of our servings of grains in their whole forms. In some cases, whole-grain processed foods contain food additives, sodium, and sweeteners. Ingredients like those may cancel out the benefit you get from the whole grain.

And grains have a lower glycemic index (GI) in their whole form than they do in their processed form. That means they're digested more slowly, so they don't cause your blood-sugar levels to spike. Steel-cut oats, for example, have a lower GI than instant oatmeal. Bulgur, or cracked wheat, has a lower GI than whole-wheat bread.

3. Eat healthy foods you like. A 2016 study from Baylor University's Hankamer School of Business found that even people with little self-control can set themselves up for healthy eating success if they switch their attention from what researchers called "avoidance" foods to "approach" foods.

Don't try to force-feed yourself something healthy that you hate (such as kale) in place of something you love (cake).

HOW TO WORK WHOLE GRAINS INTO YOUR DIET

Cooking whole grains takes a while, but they can be made in big batches and refrigerated so that you can use them in meals all week. Cooked whole grains freeze very well, too. Freeze single servings and they'll be at the ready for meals. You can use them in a variety of ways. Toss them with beans and vegetables, add them to soups or salads, incorporate them into muffin and cookie batter, or serve them as a side dish. If you like oatmeal for breakfast, try a porridge made with amaranth, barley, or millet for a change of pace. Many grains are high in protein, so they can replace meat if you're trying to cut back. Combine quinoa with mashed chickpeas for a tasty burger.

"Seek out yummy healthy foods — such as strawberries — and you might find that after enjoying a big bowl of fresh berries you no longer want that chocolate cake," says Meredith David, Ph.D., lead author of the Baylor University study.

And you can make a small snack more satisfying:

A study by Cornell University's Food and Brand Lab found that if you eat just a quarter of your usual amount (two *Hershey's Kisses,* say, instead of eight), then do something distracting for 15 minutes (take a walk), you'll feel just as satisfied as if you'd eaten the full amount.

4. Get the basics. Calories, protein, fats, and carbs are the building blocks of a healthy diet. Here's what you need to know:

- **COUNT ON CALORIES.** Yes, they *do* count. The basic formula for losing weight has not changed. To shed pounds, consume fewer calories than you burn (through everyday activities and planned exercise including strength training). How many calories do you really need? Here are guidelines from the National Institutes of Health.

APPROXIMATE # DAILY CALORIES	WOMEN	MEN
Extremely active	2,200	2,800
Moderately active	1,800	2,200–2,400
Sedentary	1,600	2,000–2,200

- **GO LEAN WITH PROTEIN.** On average, women need about 46 grams a day, men 56 grams. Just keep it lean. Enjoy salmon (29 grams of protein in 4 ounces); poultry (35 grams in 4 ounces); low-fat Greek yogurt (1 cup has 20 grams of protein); nut butter (1 tablespoon has 3.5 to 9.4 grams of protein).

Researchers found that for every 20-gram increase in "protecting" protein like beans and chicken per day, stroke risk was lowered by 20 percent. That's the amount in ⅓ cup of kidney beans or a ¼ of a chicken breast. Red meat is a protein, but it offers NO protection from stroke.

Eat *THIS* Protecting proteins

• **GET THE RIGHT AMOUNT OF THE RIGHT FATS.** The latest dietary guidelines from the government recommend keeping the calories coming from saturated fats to less than 10 percent. Avoid trans fats and focus on good-for-you fats like nuts and extra-virgin olive oil, both of which are good sources of unsaturated fat

Researchers found that when the healthy, unsaturated fats in olive oil and nuts combine with vegetables such as spinach and celery, chemical reactions occur that inhibit an enzyme that affects blood-vessel width.

Eat *THIS* Greens plus olive oil

The result: Wider blood vessels and lower blood pressure. All the more reason to use olive-oil dressing on your next salad.

• **CHOOSE COMPLEX CARBS.** When it comes to carbs, the best strategy is to focus on complex carbs like fruits, veggies, legumes, and whole-grain items. They're nutritious, satiating, and full of fiber. Avoid refined carbs with added sugar and those with white flour. Aim for taking in 45-65% of your total daily calories from complex carbs.

4 YUMMY THINGS YOU CAN EAT...BUT MIGHT HAVE THOUGHT YOU SHOULDN'T

When you ask yourself "Should I Eat This?" you may have some preconceived notions. There are some foods that you may avoid because of long-standing myths. Clearing up the confusion can make smart eating easier and more enjoyable.

1. Chicken skin

MYTH: You should take the skin off chicken before you cook it.

TRUTH: Removing the skin doesn't save you much saturated fat. This advice dates back to a time when all things fatty were considered unhealthy.

Yes, the skin contains saturated fat, but it has more of the unsaturated kind. A 3½ ounce roasted chicken breast with the skin has about 8 grams of fat, only 2 of which are saturated.

Taking the skin off saves you about 50 calories and 1 gram of saturated fat. If you're eating several pieces, those calories and fat will add up, but if you practice portion control, you can enjoy the extra flavor from perfectly crisped skin.

2. White vegetables

MYTH: White vegetables have little nutritional value.

TRUTH: The compounds that give broccoli and kale those vivid colors have antioxidant (disease-fighting) benefits. But paler veggies such as cauliflower and turnips deserve kudos too. Advice to "eat the rainbow" emerged in the 1980s when experts

were trying to get people to eat a wider variety of vegetables —
beyond the then-standard white potatoes and corn.

Cauliflower and turnips are part of the powerhouse group of
cruciferous vegetables, which also counts broccoli and kale as
members. They're high in compounds called glucosinolates, which
may have a protective role against cancer.

3. Peanut butter

MYTH: Peanut butter is too fattening to be healthy.

TRUTH: Only if you overdo it. With 94 calories and 8
grams of fat per tablespoon, peanut butter warrants
some restraint when you're slathering it on your toast or apple.

But you get a lot of nutrition for those calories, including protein,
fiber, and "good" fat.

When buying peanut butter, consider buying the stir-in type where
the oil settles on the top. That oil comes from the peanuts and
contains healthy monounsaturated fats that can help lower "bad"
(LDL) cholesterol levels and may even help some people keep off
pounds without having to strictly monitor calories.

4. Pasta

MYTH: Pasta is a fattening, diet-busting carb.

TRUTH: Pasta is a convenient, inexpensive food that's
not necessarily "fattening." In fact, pasta made from durum wheat
(semolina), has a higher protein content than most other types of pasta.

Pasta doesn't have to be off-limits even if you are trying to lose
weight. An analysis of studies published in *JAMA* found that
low-carb diets and low-fat diets (which tend to be higher in carbs)
were equally effective for weight loss. Whole grains are the
preferred choice, but there is some room in your diet for regular
white pasta.

START THE DAY RIGHT WITH CEREAL

The best breakfast in a bowl. Expert advice on how to choose a nutritious cereal.

Cereal, that old familiar breakfast staple, is less popular than it once was. That's in part because many consumers consider it to be low in protein, high in sugar, and too processed to be healthful according to the market research firm Mintel.

Although that's true of many cereals, plenty are nutritious. Plus it's quick and convenient and can be an efficient way to get many essential nutrients all at once, says Ronni Chernoff, Ph.D., director of the Arkansas Geriatric Education Collaborative. For breakfast, she recommends covering four bases: fruit, protein, a complex carbohydrate, and dairy. Have a whole-grain cereal with milk topped with fruit to hit all four.

These 4 tips can help you choose a good cereal:

1. *Pick a whole grain.* Look for a 100-percent whole-grain claim on the box, or read the ingredients list to be sure all grains are whole, such as whole wheat or whole-grain oats. Whole grains are a great source of fiber.

Having fiber for breakfast means "you're not going to be having a hunger attack midmorning," says Emily Dhurandhar, Ph.D., an assistant professor of kinesiology at Texas Tech University.

2. *Suss out the sugars.* Even a whole-grain cereal can be a poor pick if it contains too much added sugar. *Kellogg's Frosted Mini-Wheats*, for example, is made from 100-percent whole-grain wheat and has 6 grams of fiber per serving, but it also has 11 grams of sugars, almost 3 teaspoons. Compare that with *Post Spoon Size Shredded Wheat*, which has 0 grams of sugars per serving. (The American Heart Association recommends no more than 25 grams of added sugars per day for women, 36 grams for men.)

"If you want it sweet, add fruit or even a teaspoon of sugar if you need to," says Maxine Siegel, R.D., who heads the food-testing lab at Consumer Reports. "But if you're going to buy a sweetened cereal, choose one with no more than 8 grams of sugars per serving."

3. *Pay attention to protein.* Having protein in the morning may help keep blood sugar steady and aid weight control. Cereals usually have 3 to 4 grams of protein per serving;

3 GOOD CEREAL PICKS

Consumer Reports rated several brands of cereal for taste and nutrition. These performed well in our analysis:

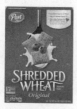

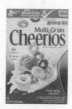

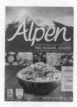

High Fiber
POST SHREDDED
WHEAT
Serving: 1 cup
170 calories |
0 g sugars | 6 g fiber
6 g protein

Sweet Cereal
CHEERIOS
MULTI GRAIN
Serving: 1 cup
110 calories | 6 g
sugars | 3 g fiber
2 g protein

High Protein
ALPEN MUESLI
NO SUGAR ADDED
Serving: ⅔ cup
210 calories | 8 g
sugars | 6 g fiber
7 g protein

some contain 6 or more grams. Pour on cow's milk, and you'll add about 3 to 4 grams per ½ cup. Some soy milks have that much protein, but almond and coconut milks have hardly any. Or top your cereal with plain yogurt, which will add about 4 grams per ½ cup.

4. *Watch your portions.* In a test, Siegel's team asked consumers to fill a bowl with the amount of cereal they would typically serve themselves. About 92 percent poured too much—24 to 282 percent more than the serving size on the box. "A double helping of cereal can give you more fiber and protein, but it can also bump up the calories, sugars, and sodium," Siegel says. So grab your favorite bowl, pour out the amount you usually eat, and measure it. Then do the math so you know what you're really eating.

CHAPTER TWO

SHOP

Eat *THIS*
to control your weight

I f you check the nutrition label of almonds, you may find a relatively high calorie count and be dissuaded from eating them in spite of the health benefits. But now, scientists have found that the body doesn't actually absorb all the calories in almonds. There are about 170 calories in an ounce of almonds, but research shows only about 129 calories are retained by the body. An ounce is about 23 almonds.

IN THIS CHAPTER:

DO YOU NEED TO BUY ORGANIC OR NOT?

How to shop smarter *(and healthier)* at the supermarket.

As a general rule, organic food costs more than conventional food, but is it worth the extra money? Here's a guide to which organic choices will provide the most immediate benefit and when you should, or shouldn't, buy organic.

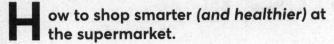

BEEF   *Importance of buying organic:* Medium to high

Why: Grassfed and organic beef have nutritional benefits

Organic cattle are not raised with routine antibiotics. The widespread use of those drugs in food animals is contributing to a rise in antibiotic-resistant bacteria.

For optimal nutritional benefits, look for organic meat that's also labeled "American Grassfed Approved" or "USDA Process Verified Grassfed." That guarantees that the animal was raised on a diet of 99 percent grass and forage and had seasonal access to a pasture. Studies suggest that meat from such animals might provide more health benefits than meat from animals fattened on a conventional diet of grain.

POULTRY   *Importance of buying organic:* Medium to high

Why: To discourage the use of antibiotics and questionable feed

Organic poultry is raised almost always without the routine use of antibiotics. And organic birds can't be fed arsenic drugs or poultry litter — a mixture of droppings, spilled feed, and feathers.

DAIRY | *Importance of buying organic:* Medium to high

Why: Nutritional benefits

Organic dairy cows are not treated with growth hormones and must eat an organic diet that doesn't contain animal by-products.

Research has found that organic milk contains about 60 percent more heart-healthy omega-3 fatty acids than nonorganic versions, a benefit that also extends to cheese and yogurt.

PRODUCE | *Importance of buying organic:* It depends

Why: You often have a low-risk conventional option

Experts at Consumer Reports believe that organic is always the best choice for your health, the environment, and the people who grow our food. And organic produce is always low-risk when it comes to pesticide residues. While the risks of pesticides are real, the myriad health benefits of fruits and vegetables are too. That's why we remind you that while *organic* is best, don't skip conventionally grown produce.

A 2012 study estimated that increasing fruit and vegetable consumption could prevent 20,000 cancer cases annually — but 10 cases of cancer per year could be attributed to consumption of pesticides from the additional produce.

Another study found that people who ate produce at least

three times per day had a lower risk of stroke, hypertension, and death from cardiovascular disease.

Your primary goal is to eat a diet rich in fruits and vegetables — ideally five or more servings a day — and they don't all have to be organically grown.

The relative risk from pesticides on conventional produce varies from very low to very high, depending on the type of produce and on the country where it's grown.

The differences can be dramatic. For instance, eating one serving of green beans from the U.S. is 200 times riskier than eating a serving of U.S. grown broccoli.

10 FOODS YOU SHOULD ALWAYS BUY ORGANIC — no matter where they're grown:

Peaches	Cranberries	Hot Peppers
Tangerines	Green Beans	Sweet Potatoes
Nectarines	Sweet Bell Peppers	Carrots
Strawberries		

10 FOODS THAT YOU DON'T HAVE TO BUY ORGANIC — if they are grown in:

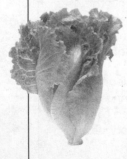

Apples ....New Zealand
Avocado...Chile, Mexico, Peru
Broccoli .... U.S., Mexico
Cherries...U.S.
Cherry Tomatoes..U.S.
Grapefruit...U.S.
Grapes................................Chile, Mexico, Peru, U.S.
Lettuce .... Mexico, U.S.
Oranges .... Chile, South Africa, U.S.
Pears..Argentina, U.S.

Eat *THESE:* In our blind taste tests, we found the items below to be tops in their category for both nutrition and taste. You might like to try them.

Almond butter	• 365 Everyday Value [Whole Foods] Almond Butter Creamy • Kirkland Signature [Costco] Almond Butter Creamy • Trader Joe's Raw Almond Butter Creamy
Frozen appetizers	• Trader Joe's Chicken Gyoza Potstickers • Saffron Road Crispy Samosas with Vegetables • Whole Foods Market™ Artichoke, Kale & Swiss Chard Bites
Coffee	• Counter Culture La Golondrina (bold beans) • La Colombe Ethiopia-Yirgz • Dunkin' Donuts 100% Colombian (ground beans)
Alternative pasta *(pastas made with lentils, chickpeas or quinoa blends)*	• Ancient Harvest POW! Red Lentil Rotini • Explore Cuisine Organic Chickpea Fusilli • Hodgson Mill UltraGrain® Penne With Quinoa
Veggie burgers	• Morningstar Farms Garden Veggie • Boca All American Flame Grilled • Amy's Light in Sodium California

Eat *THIS*

Salmon

When shopping for salmon, you may have wondered if canned salmon is as good for you as fresh. Well, consider this: A USDA study found slightly higher levels of good-for-you omega-3s in canned pink and red salmon compared to fresh salmon. Canned salmon has other merits too: A 3.5-ounce serving delivers almost as much calcium as a glass of skim milk, if you eat the soft little bones.

SUPERMARKET MEALS

Prepared foods are now the rage in supermarkets. Convenience may have fueled this trend, but what's keeping it going is a desire for meals we think are healthier than traditional takeout or dinners from the frozen-food aisle.

3 THINGS YOU SHOULD KNOW *BEFORE* YOU PICK UP YOUR NEXT SUPERMARKET MEAL.

Consumer Reports wanted to find out whether this burgeoning breed of convenience food is actually fresh and healthful. Our nutrition experts and secret shoppers scanned the prepared-food cases at six major supermarket chains in the Northeast.

We investigated where the food was prepared and how the food was prepared, and we analyzed the food in a laboratory for calories, fat, saturated fat, sodium, and— for foods expected to contain it—fiber.

Our testing and analysis revealed some surprising findings:

1. *"Freshly made" doesn't always mean fresh ingredients.* Not all stores promise that the dishes they sell are fresh and not processed. But that's certainly the implication; by going to a bustling counter with chef-like personnel, you might think you're getting a meal that's something close to homemade in the traditional sense of the word.

But you'd be wrong to assume that there are always cooks in

the back peeling and mashing potatoes or dipping chicken cutlets into egg and breadcrumbs. In fact, only about half of the dishes we purchased for our tests were made on the premises according to the store clerks who were quizzed by our secret shoppers.

None of the supermarkets we went to made every prepared dish they sold in house. What's more, our investigation revealed that some dishes weren't even prepared in the same ZIP code as the store.

"In-store preparation" — a kitchen in every location — carries high costs. As a result, those stores that make dishes onsite charge accordingly.

So where does most of the prepared food sold in supermarkets come from? Some chains use centralized kitchens to prepare big batches of ready-to-serve dishes such as soup, then deliver them to stores.

Others "provide meal solutions that consumers perceive to be fresh but in fact have been delivered frozen (to the supermarket) and are reheated in the store 'kitchen'" according to a report from the consulting and research firms A.T. Kearney and Technomic.

Neither option produces dishes that are necessarily free of preservatives or other ingredients you'll find in processed food. The mashed potatoes we bought from two supermarkets, for instance, contained sodium benzoate, a preservative, and disodium pyrophosphate to maintain color.

Sometimes, the fresh meals were actually made with packaged processed foods. The creamy sauce that topped one turkey meatloaf, for example, wasn't the supermarket chef's recipe. The counterperson told our shopper that it was actually a brand of bottled poppyseed salad dressing.

Is any of this actually harmful for consumers? Not necessarily. But many people try to minimize the processed foods in their diet, sometimes for health reasons such as a sensitivity to preservatives. And they might assume — not unreasonably — that the dish they bought is made from fresh ingredients.

MAKING THE MOST OF SUPERMARKET MEALS
From Amy Keating, Consumer Reports Registered Dietitian

1. Buy prepared foods to eat today or soon after.
You want them to be as fresh as possible, so plan to store them in the fridge for no more than three or four days, max. (That's true for leftover prepared meals too.)

2. When shopping, pick up prepared food last so the cold items stay cold and the hot items stay hot. Buy hot food only if you plan to eat it within 2 hours, making sure to keep it at least at 140°F. Otherwise, it's better to buy food that needs refrigerating, then reheat it to at least 165°F.

3. The idea is that prepared food is an alternative to cooking at home, so it should contain the kind of ingredients you cook with, such as fresh vegetables and spices, and it shouldn't have a lot of added salt. If something is smothered in gravy or slick with oil, for example, it's probably not a healthy choice.

4. You can stretch a prepared food dish to save money as well as calories, fat, and sodium. For example, serve a prepared side dish from the deli counter over fresh greens from the produce section.

Common allergens like nuts and eggs often have to be disclosed, but federal regulations don't always mandate that stores provide an ingredients list unless the food has a health claim such as "low fat."

Most of the stores we went to provided that information. But some lists were missing ingredients. The salad dressing on one store's turkey meatloaf didn't appear on the ingredients list, nor did the clearly visible avocado in some samples of spicy tuna roll. Omissions such as these could pose a problem for people with allergies to less common ingredients, or those who avoid certain ingredients because they're high in fat, calories, or sodium, says Amy Keating, R.D., a dietitian at Consumer Reports who oversaw our testing.

2. Pass the salt, again and again and again. Most of the sodium in our diet comes from salt added to processed and restaurant foods. But our testing revealed that there's loads of sodium hiding in the dishes you find in the prepared-foods department, Keating says.

We found one store's mini-turkey meatloaves to be mini salt licks with 891 milligrams in 6 ounces. And who would guess that a cup of delicate lemon orzo was a salt bomb, with 938 milligrams per serving? That's about 40 percent of the daily recommended limit of 2,300 milligrams per day. How about the vegetarian eggplant rollatini (635 milligrams) or spicy tuna rolls (834 milligrams in 6 ounces)?

The health consequences of overdosing on sodium are serious. Too much boosts the risk of high blood pressure, which in turn raises the risk of heart disease and stroke.

3. *Stores can stonewall on nutritional information.*
Even more of a concern was that when nutritional information was available from a store, it didn't always match our lab's findings.

One store, for example, claimed its turkey meatloaf had 7 grams of fat, but our findings revealed an average of 18 grams per serving. We also found wide variations in some nutrients in the same dishes from store to store. Our three samples of one supermarket's chicken marsala, for example, ranged from 359 milligrams of sodium per 6 ounces to 1,003 milligrams. The amount of fat in the tortellini and sundried tomato salad from another was 18 to 29 grams per cup.

RATINGS: SUPERMARKET-PREPARED FOODS

In a Consumer Reports supermarket survey, almost 63,000 subscribers reported on 111,000 shopping trips, giving their opinions on measures from produce quality to cleanliness. That is reflected in the OVERALL SCORE. We also rate consumer satisfaction with the quality of prepared food in the STORE-PREPARED FOOD SCORES.

STORE	OVERALL SCORE	STORE-PREPARED FOOD SCORES
TOP SCORES		
Wegmans	90	⌃⌃
Publix	87	⌃⌃
Costco	84	⌃⌃
The Fresh Market	83	⌃⌃
Whole Foods Market	81	⌃
Trader Joe's	87	⌃
Fareway Stores	85	⌃
Market Basket (Northeast)	85	⌃
Raley's	84	⌃
Sprouts Farmers Market	83	⌃
Hy-Vee	82	⌃
H-E-B	82	⌃
Fry's	81	⌃
Harris Teeter	81	⌃
King Soopers	80	⌃
Hannaford	79	⌃
Dillons	78	⌃
Schnucks	78	⌃
Country Market	78	⌃
QFC	77	⌃
Ingles	77	⌃
Marsh	77	⌃
Big Y	76	⌃
BOTTOM SCORES		
Food 4 Less	78	⌄
Target/Super Target	75	⌄
Food Lion	73	⌄
Tops Markets	67	⌄
Walmart Supercenter	64	⌄
Aldi	81	⌄⌄

7 FOOD LABELS THAT CAN FOOL YOU

Is it really good for you? You see a lot of nutrition buzzwords on food labels, but they don't always mean what you think.

When you're grocery shopping, here's a good rule of thumb: Be wary of the healthy-sounding words on food packages.

Almost 70 percent of consumers in a new survey of 1,000 people from the Consumer Reports National Research Center said they use the front-of-package information when deciding whether to buy processed foods for the first time — but it's probably not helping them make better choices.

"From the perspective of the average consumer, front-of-package claims are sometimes misleading and may lead people to make unhealthy food purchases," says Kristin Kirkpatrick, M.S., R.D., L.D., manager of wellness nutrition services at the Cleveland Clinic Wellness Institute.

Many terms and phrases aren't regulated by the USDA, and some can be misinterpreted — by implying a health attribute that's not exactly true.

7 label claims that may not mean what you think they do:

1. *The label says "LIGHT IN SODIUM," but:* This phrase can easily be confused with "low sodium," a term the FDA defines as containing 140 milligrams of sodium or less per serving.

But "light in sodium" means that a product has 50 percent or less of the sodium in the manufacturer's regular version —

so it can still be fairly salty. If the standard food is very high in sodium, that label isn't helpful.

Take *Pacific Organic Creamy Tomato Soup*, for example. The regular version has 750 milligrams of sodium per 1-cup serving. The "light in sodium" version has 380 milligrams per cup. Have that with a few saltines, and you've consumed about 20 percent of the maximum amount of sodium you should have in a day.

2. The label says "SIMPLY MADE," but:

Usually, products with this claim have a short ingredients list, but the term isn't regulated. And short doesn't equal healthy. *Simply Made Keebler Butter Cookies* have 70 calories each and a fair amount of fat and sugars.

3. The label says "LIGHTLY SWEETENED," but:

The FDA has a definition for this term for canned fruit but not for other foods. For example, *Fiber One Honey Clusters* cereal has "lightly sweetened" written on the front of its box, but a single cup has 9 grams of sugars, about 2 teaspoons. The American Heart Association suggests getting just 6 to 9 teaspoons of added sugars per day.

You may also see "touch of" honey or brown sugar on a package. Products with that wording can still be pretty sugary. *Quaker® Oatmeal Squares* cereal, with "a hint of honey" on the box, has 9 grams of sugars per ½ cup, for example — the same amount as in a ¾ cup serving of *Kellogg's Special K Chocolatey Delight*.

4. The label says "WHOLE GRAIN," but: "Whole-grain"

foods can also have refined flour. One example is *Cheez-It® Whole Grain* crackers.

These crackers contain whole-wheat flour but also refined flour. That leaves you with just 1 gram of fiber per serving (27 crackers), 8 grams of fat, and 250 milligrams of sodium.

If you want whole grain, look for the words "100-percent whole grain" on the package and check ingredients lists. A whole-grain flour should be the first ingredient, and the product should have no enriched flours at all.

5. *The label says "NATURAL," but:* The use of the word "natural" can be a deceptive marketing ploy to reel in unaware consumers. People are led to believe it is the same as "organic," and it is not.

In fact, for processed foods, that term has no clear meaning and is not regulated by any agency. Don't be duped by "natural" labels that currently aren't backed by meaningful standards.

 For example, *Del Monte Fruit Naturals* snacks contain natural fruits such as peaches, pears, and cherries. But they also contain artificial preservatives made from industrial chemicals: potassium sorbate and sodium benzoate.

6. *The label says "NO NITRATES ADDED," but:* Meat with this label may not have been cured with synthetic nitrates, but it may have been cured with concentrated nitrates from vegetables such as celery and onion. The curing chemistry is the same no matter where the nitrate comes from. The World Health Organization classifies artificial nitrates as "probably carcinogenic to humans." Check ingredients lists for celery juice or celery powder — which act as nitrates and carry the same risks as artificial nitrates.

7. *The label says "REAL," but:* This does not mean chemical-free or unprocessed. For example, *Hormel Real Crumbled Bacon* has smoke flavoring, preservatives, sugar, and salts.

"GOOD" BUTTERY SPREADS AREN'T NECESSARILY GOOD FOR YOU

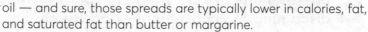

Some brands of buttery spreads boast that they're made with olive oil or canola oil — and sure, those spreads are typically lower in calories, fat, and saturated fat than butter or margarine.

But that does not mean they have the same nutritional profile as the oils themselves. Most buttery spreads are a blend of the featured oil and other vegetable oils.

And all spreads — even those made with olive oil or yogurt — contain trans or saturated fat.

I Can't Believe It's Not Butter Light has palm and palm kernel oils, which can be as bad for your heart as partially hydrogenated oil, if not worse.

People who got the bulk of their fat from palm oil, palm kernel, or coconut oil for about five weeks saw their LDL ("bad") cholesterol rise just as much as people on a high partially hydrogenated oil diet according to an analysis by the New York Department of Health and Mental Hygiene.

TIP: *Look for products made of healthier canola or olive oil instead of palm or palm kernel oil.*

Don't Eat *THIS*

Banana chips

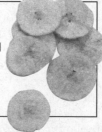

Yes, they're made from good-for-you bananas, but they're usually fried in coconut or palm oil, unhealthy sources of saturated fat. There can be up to 210 calories and 13 grams of fat per serving.

21 WAYS TO SAVE TIME AND MONEY AT THE SUPERMARKET

Supermarkets are changing to suit a more discriminating consumer — and online grocers are coming on strong. Here, how to save money and still make healthy choices.

Consumer Reports asked experts as well as our Facebook followers for their best time- and money-saving food shopping tips. Pick a few of these tactics to try in the coming weeks; you could shave up to 40 percent off your bill.

1. *Look high and low for best deals.* You'll find the lower-cost generic versions of cereal, cake mixes, paper goods, and other high-turnover staples on the very lowest and highest supermarket shelves. Retailers can charge manufacturers a fee to be at eye level.

2. *Try discount apps for savings and freebies.* Two we like are *Ibotta* and *Flipp*. Both coordinate your store loyalty cards with current discounts and coupons. With *Flipp*, you scan the app with the market's checkout scanner to apply savings at the point of sale. With *Ibotta*, you select rebates in the app and photograph your receipts to import savings to an *Ibotta* account. Savings are transferred to a payment app, such as *PayPal*, or a gift card.

3. *Outsmart temptation with a GPS.* Before you drive to someplace you've never been, you should probably tap the address into a smartphone or GPS. The same concept applies to shopping: If your destination is "healthy," you need to make the right turns to arrive there. The supermarket can be a tricky thoroughfare, and you need directions. Some store loyalty club apps let you locate items by aisle, which can help you avoid crisscrossing aisles — and avoid temptations. At major chains, the *Flipp* app can do the same.

4. Yes, do the math. Unit price shelf stickers under each product can help you compare. But if the store doesn't have the stickers, use your smartphone's calculator. Divide the price by the number of units in each package you're comparing. If, say, one soda's price is per fluid ounce and the other's is per liter, ask Google how many ounces are in a liter and do the conversions.

5. Ask for a rain check. When a sale item is sold out, ask a store employee for a rain check — a paper IOU — that you can use like a coupon when the item's in stock. "I've saved hundreds of dollars this way," says Jeanette Pavini, a consumer savings analyst at *Quotient*, which is based in Mountain View, California, and runs the shopping app and website Coupons.com.

6. Remember, store brands may be better than brand names. Consumer Reports' trained tasters have found store brands with quality equal — or *superior* — to that of brand-name items, at prices usually 15 to 30 percent lower. That's because generics are sometimes made by the same companies that make the big-brand foods. *Trader Joe's* was a standout for its store brands in our survey. In past taste tests of 57 store brands, we found that 33 were as good as or better than the comparable name brand, including those in the product categories of frozen shrimp, roasted cashews, cranberry juice cocktail, ketchup, maple syrup, mayonnaise, frozen mixed vegetables, shredded mozzarella, and vanilla ice cream.

7. Use a cash-back card. Consumer Reports found great potential savings from the *American Express Blue Cash Preferred® Card*, which pays back 6 percent on the first $6,000 in groceries each year as well as 3 percent on gas and department-store purchases and 1 percent on other purchases. It also returns $150 if you spend $1,000 in the first three months. That means if you spend $200 monthly on gas, $500 on groceries, $100 on department store buys, and $300 on other items, you would save $583 in the first year of card ownership and $1,449 in the first three years, even factoring in the $95 annual fee.

8. *Inspect store circulars. Even if you do it digitally.*
Only 46 percent of millennial shoppers in our recent survey said they read store circulars for weekly sales, compared with 51 percent of Generation Xers and 63 percent of Baby Boomers. Most circulars are online, making the task of checking them pretty painless even for the digital-first crowd.

9. *Embrace coupons.* Find stores that double or even
triple manufacturers' paper coupons. Certain retailers do it every day or week, others less regularly. In the Northeast, *Stop & Shop* doubles manufacturers' paper coupons every day. *HI-LO*, in Georgia, North Carolina, and South Carolina, doubles coupons with a value of 60 cents or less every day, unless noted otherwise at the individual store. (With both chains, other restrictions apply.)

10. *Do a pantry inventory.* Americans throw away about
a quarter of the food and beverages they buy, at a cost of up to $2,275 annually for the average family of four, says the Natural Resources Defense Council. Use the free USDA FoodKeeper app for guidelines on how to store foods.

Or do as Maggie Pallan, a professional chef in Las Vegas, does. She maintains a spreadsheet of what she has at home to avoid buying duplicates. "I treat my home grocery shopping the same as my business," she says.

11. *Get senior discounts.* Several chains, including *HI-LO*, *Harris Teeter*, *Hy-Vee*, and *Publix*, offer 5 percent discounts, either on specific days and/or when you present a special store ID card. The *Fred Meyer* discount is 10 percent. In some cases, you must be at least 60 to qualify.

12. *Weigh bagged produce — you may find a bonus.* Prebagged produce is usually cheaper by the pound than individual pieces. Use the produce scale to compare bags because they're not uniform in weight. A Consumer Reports reporter found 3-pound bags of red delicious apples at a *Stop & Shop* near our Yonkers headquarters weighing from 3.06 to 3.36 pounds, a 10 percent bonus.

DON'T shop at the busiest times

According to a survey by the Time Use Institute, a consulting company, the busiest time on weekdays is from 4 p.m. to 5 p.m.

The least busy is before 8 a.m. and after 6 p.m. On weekends, the peak shopping time is from 11 a.m. to noon.

13. *Buy in bulk — even if you don't have storage space.* When 10 cans of your favorite soup go on sale for $10, load up. If you don't have room to store that many, check the promotion wording to see whether you're required to buy all 10 for the discount.

14. *Track prices.* For a few weeks, record prices of the items you buy the most. Once you know where to find the best prices for specific goods, you can stock up when a true price drop happens. Price-tracking also helps you see when a "10 packages for $10" sale really is a sale and not just a come-on.

15. *Find online bargains — especially for these 4 foods.* Online services often waive the delivery fee or give discounts for first-time customers. Even with the delivery charge, buying online can help you uncover savings for certain kinds of foods, notably snack bars, specialty diet food, coffee, and pasta, says Sam Gagliardi, head of e-commerce at *IRI Worldwide*, a market research company in Chicago. Online vendors such as *AmazonFresh* often offer prices up to half off regional grocery chains' prices because they match *Walmart* and warehouse clubs' national prices, Gagliardi explains.

16. *Shop the drugstore — for items you might not think of as drugstore items.* Convenience stores, drugstores, and even gas station mini-marts can sometimes beat prices at traditional markets for staples such as milk and eggs. Just be mindful of expiration dates. Food that has outlived its expiration date can still be sold, assuming it is "wholesome and fit for consumption" and not dangerous to consumers according to the FDA.

17. *Beware of prepared foods — they can be unhealthy and pricey.* A 2016 Consumer Reports investigation found that supermarket-prepared items might not be made in the store and might have preservatives and excess salt. And sure, ready-made items such as cranberry couscous and lemon orzo with pine nuts can tempt when you're in a rush. But for simple items — say, sautéed greens — home prep can cost about half the price and take less than half an hour of work, our staff food experts say. A home-prep bonus: fewer unnecessary ingredients.

18. *Look for "as-is items" that are good to go.* The overripe bananas you'll find at a discount could be perfect for homemade banana bread. Learn where stores have their clearance sections, says Annette Economides, who with her husband, Steve, runs the website MoneySmartFamily.com. *Publix* stores, for instance, place clearance items on a dedicated rack.

19. *Bring your own bags.* This might make loading take a little longer but could also save you money at stores that charge for bags, as more and more municipalities require them to do. You'll also help reduce plastic waste in the environment.

And be sure to keep your reusable bags clean. Store bags in the cleanest area of the car and launder or wipe them down with hot, soapy water at least once per month, or after each use if they were used to transport raw meat or seafood.

20. *Shop on "cheaper" weekdays.* Certain items are cheaper on weekdays, when stores seek to clear inventory, says Bryan Leach, founder and CEO of the shopping app *Ibotta*. Consumer data collected through his app show the best and worst days to shop for various items:

- **Monday** for best prices on ice cream and beauty products. Beer is 9% cheaper on Monday (and most costly on Saturday).

- **Tuesday** for best prices on wine.

- **Wednesday** for best prices on produce. (Monday is the most expensive day for produce.)

- **Thursday** for best prices on cleaning products.

- **Friday** for best prices on snacks.

21. *Use your freezer right – you might save $2,000 a year.* Freezing large quantities of sale and seasonal food saves the average family of four $2,000 per year, Annette Economides maintains. "Why pay $4 a pound for blueberries in winter when you can thaw the ones you bought in summer for much less?" she asks. The Economideses even freeze milk and cheese. Every 30 to 60 days they check the freezer and build menus based on what's there.

WHY YOU SHOULD FILL YOUR SHOPPING CART WITH POTASSIUM-RICH FOODS

When it comes to dietary strategies to lower blood pressure, sodium gets all the attention. But too little potassium could be just as important as too much salt. "When you get enough potassium, it helps your body excrete sodium," says Angie Murad, R.D., a nutritionist at the Mayo Clinic Healthy Living Program. "That eases tension in the blood vessel walls, which can help lower blood pressure." The mineral also helps blood vessels relax independent of the role it plays in sodium balance.

The recommended daily dose of potassium is 4,700 mg. But according to a study in *The American Journal of Clinical Nutrition*, fewer than 2 percent of Americans consume that much. Having at least eight servings of fruits and vegetables daily is ideal. "But if you just focus on eating fruits and vegetables with every meal and for snacks, you will easily get enough," Murad says. (See Pump up the potassium, page 154).

11 GOOD SOURCES OF POTASSIUM

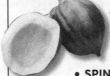

- **ACORN SQUASH**
  1 cup, cubed, 896 mg
- **SPINACH**
  1 cup, cooked, 839 mg
- **BAKED POTATO**
  1 small, w/skin, 738 mg
- **SALMON**
  5 ounces, 676 mg
- **WHITE BEANS**
  ½ cup, 502 mg

- **YOGURT, LOW-FAT, PLAIN**
  1 cup, 531 mg
- **CANTALOUPE**
  1 cup, cubed, 427 mg
- **BANANA**
  1 medium, 422 mg
- **SWEET POTATO**
  1 medium, no skin, 347 mg
- **AVOCADO**
  ½ fruit, 345 mg
- **PISTACHIOS**
  ¼ cup kernels, 310 mg

CHAPTER THREE

EAT

Eat *THIS*
to keep your body young

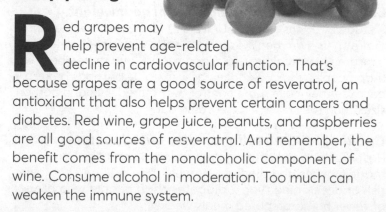

R ed grapes may help prevent age-related decline in cardiovascular function. That's because grapes are a good source of resveratrol, an antioxidant that also helps prevent certain cancers and diabetes. Red wine, grape juice, peanuts, and raspberries are all good sources of resveratrol. And remember, the benefit comes from the nonalcoholic component of wine. Consume alcohol in moderation. Too much can weaken the immune system.

IN THIS CHAPTER:

QUICK, EASY, HEALTHY RECIPES

Creating your own healthy meals can be fast and fun. Here are six delicious dishes simple enough to whip up in a snap.

Americans are eating out more than ever before. We'll spend an estimated $720 billion at restaurants this year. That's almost half of every food dollar we spend. And this shift may be having an impact on more than just our wallets. Eating at home can cut costs, and pounds — while improving your health.

Cooking at home can help control your weight.
A study by Johns Hopkins University found that people who make their own meals as infrequently as twice a week consume fewer calories, fats, and sugars, and more fiber than people who cook once per week or less. That's probably because they have more control over ingredients and portion sizes than they do when they dine out.

Cooking for yourself may also cut diabetes risk.
Research shows that people who ate 11 or more home-made lunches and dinners per week had a 12 percent lower risk of developing type 2 diabetes than people who ate six or fewer home-prepared meals weekly.

Cooking at home may help protect your heart health.
Restaurant and take-out meals are often drenched in salt. But when you eat at home you can cut your sodium intake, which may lower your risk of high blood pressure and heart disease.

Finding time to cook at home can be challenging. To make it easier, we asked the experts in our test kitchen for two days' worth of recipes for fast, filling meals. Mix and match these ideas as you like, and for your health's sake, *EAT THESE:*

Scrambled Egg and Veggie Wrap

½ red pepper, chopped

¼ onion, chopped

1 tsp olive oil

2 eggs

1 tbsp water

1 whole-wheat tortilla

1 tbsp shredded Monterey Jack cheese

½ cup spinach

Sauté red pepper and onion in olive oil until tender. Whisk eggs in bowl with water; add to veggies and cook over medium heat until eggs are completely cooked. Spoon onto whole-wheat tortilla. Top with shredded cheese and spinach; roll up.

Makes one serving; double the ingredients to serve two.

NUTRITION AT A GLANCE
Calories 370, Fat 19 g, Saturated fat 5 g,
Protein 19 g, Fiber 4 g, Sodium 310 mg

Morning Quinoa

¼ cup quinoa

½ cup skim milk

¼ tsp vanilla

¼ tsp cinnamon

¼ cup unsalted cashews

½ cup blueberries

1 tsp honey

Bring quinoa, skim milk, vanilla, and cinnamon to a boil. Simmer, covered, until quinoa is tender and liquid is absorbed, 10 to 12 minutes. Let sit for 5 minutes. Mix in cashews and blueberries. Drizzle with honey.

Makes one serving; double the ingredients to serve two.

NUTRITION AT A GLANCE
Calories 460, Fat 19 g, Saturated fat 3.5 g, Protein 16 g, Fiber 6 g, Sodium 60 mg

Easy Salad Nicoise

2 cups baby lettuce

3 oz drained light canned tuna

1 yellow pepper, thinly sliced

½ cup blanched green beans

6 grape tomatoes, halved

1 hard-boiled egg, sliced

¼ cup chickpeas

1 tbsp nicoise (or other) olives

¼ cup basil leaves

1 tbsp olive oil

2 tsp red-wine vinegar

1 tsp Dijon mustard

½ cup croutons

Top lettuce with tuna, pepper, green beans, tomatoes, egg, chickpeas, olives, and basil leaves. Toss with olive oil, vinegar, and Dijon mustard. Top with croutons.

Makes one serving; double the ingredients to serve two.

NUTRITION AT A GLANCE
Calories 510, Fat 23 g, Saturated fat 4 g,
Protein 33 g, Fiber 10 g, Sodium 640 mg

Turkey and Brie Sandwich with Apple Butter

2 tbsp apple butter

1 whole-wheat pita

3 oz roasted turkey

1 oz Brie cheese

1 apple, thinly sliced

A few leaves of red-leaf lettuce

Spread apple butter on both sides of pita. Top with roasted turkey, cheese, ½ of apple slices, and lettuce. Serve remaining apple slices on the side.

Makes one serving; double the ingredients to serve two.

NUTRITION AT A GLANCE
Calories 500, Fat 11 g, Saturated fat 5 g, Protein 39 g, Fiber 9 g, Sodium 500 mg

---

Farro with Grilled Chicken, Butternut Squash, and Kale

2 cups shredded kale

½ cup cooked farro

½ cup roasted butternut squash cubes

½ fresh pear, chopped

2 tbsp crumbled feta cheese

2 tbsp pumpkin seeds

3 oz grilled chicken cut into pieces

1 tbsp olive oil

2 tsp balsamic vinegar

½ small garlic clove, minced

Combine kale, farro, butternut squash, pear, feta cheese, and pumpkin seeds. Top with grilled chicken. Toss with olive oil, balsamic vinegar, and minced garlic.

Makes one serving; double the ingredients to serve two.

NUTRITION AT A GLANCE
Calories 640, Fat 28 g, Saturated fat 7 g,
Protein 42 g, Fiber 11 g, Sodium 260 mg

Penne with Asparagus and Peas

1 cup whole-wheat penne

½ cup asparagus pieces

¼ cup frozen peas

½ cup small-curd 2% cottage cheese

2 tsp olive oil

2 tbsp grated Parmesan cheese

Pinch each of nutmeg and black pepper

1 tbsp chopped parsley

1 tsp lemon zest

Cook penne. Add asparagus in the last 3 minutes of cooking and peas during the last minute. Drain, saving ¼ cup cooking water. Mix cottage cheese, oil, Parmesan, nutmeg, and black pepper. Stir in pasta, using reserved pasta water if needed. Top with parsley and lemon zest.

Makes one serving; double the ingredients to serve two.

NUTRITION AT A GLANCE
Calories 620, Fat 20 g, Saturated fat 5 g, Protein 35 g, Fiber 20 g, Sodium 630 mg

SUPERFOOD VS. SUPER HYPE

You may have heard them called superfoods, power foods, or miracle cures. But the research is still out on exactly how beneficial they are — and some may have a downside.

APPLE CIDER VINEGAR

THE CLAIMS:
Drinking it regularly fights bacteria, lowers cholesterol, controls blood-sugar levels, and aids weight loss. It also fights heartburn, because low acid causes heartburn, and vinegar is an acid.

THE REALITY:
It makes for a great salad dressing, but the health benefits of apple cider vinegar are overblown. Gastroenterologist William Chey, M.D. says there's no solid evidence that low acid levels lead to reflux. And Chey reports that he has treated several patients who have damaged their esophagus by overdoing it on this vinegar.

BONE BROTH

THE CLAIMS: It fights inflammation, makes skin look younger, and boosts energy.

THE REALITY: Bone broth is simply stock, which is made by simmering animal or fish bones. "While it's been used as a traditional medicine for hundreds of years, there are likely benefits, but there isn't much published research," says integrative nutritionist Robin Foroutan, M.S., R.D.N. It may help with inflammation.

COCONUT OIL

THE CLAIMS:
This saturated fat doesn't raise cholesterol levels the way other saturated fats do. It also promotes weight loss and prevents Alzheimer's disease.

THE REALITY:
Some small studies suggest that coconut oil may be less unhealthy than other saturated fats, such as those in red meat and full-fat dairy products.

Adding a small amount of coconut oil to your diet may be reasonable if you use it to replace other oils or fats, but its purported health benefits haven't been proved. And like other oils, it contains about 120 calories per tablespoon.

THE FOUNTAIN OF YOUTH DIET?

You don't have to totally give up meat to get the health rewards of a veggie lifestyle. A semi-vegetarian diet can be totally rewarding.

A strong body of research supports the idea that a plant-centric diet can boost your health; decrease your risk of heart disease, type 2 diabetes, and certain cancers; and help you stay at a healthy weight.

It can even lengthen your life according to a study in *JAMA Internal Medicine* that tracked more than 70,000 people.

But for many, life without steak, barbecued chicken, or pork tacos doesn't sound so appealing. Fortunately, you don't have to make an either/or choice.

"Just making a shift to a more plant-based diet can offer significant health benefits," says Reed Mangels, Ph.D., R.D., an adjunct associate professor of nutrition at the University of Massachusetts Amherst.

Research shows that flexitarians — those who make plant foods the star of their diet, with meat, fish, dairy, and eggs playing a supporting role — are healthier than frequent meat eaters in categories such as colon cancer and heart-disease risk and overall mortality.

THE POWER OF PLANTS

The main advantages of a mostly vegetarian diet seem to be more related to the foods you're eating lots of (vegetables, fruits, whole grains, beans, nuts) rather than those you're eating less of (meat).

"When you base your meals on plant foods, you're packing your diet with the fiber, vitamins, minerals, and healthy fats that most Americans don't get enough of," says Sharon Palmer, R.D., author of *The Plant-Powered Diet*. Plant-based diets are also full of phyto-chemicals, compounds that help keep many of your body's systems running smoothly.

Eat *THESE*

- **BERRIES.** They contain anthocyanins to help protect vision.

- **CARROTS AND CANTALOUPE.** They contain carotenoids to help protect against cancer and heart disease.

- **GARLIC.** It contains sulfur compounds that may help inhibit blood clots and reduce cholesterol levels.

SEMI-VEGETARIAN PERKS

How much meat can you eat and still get the benefits of a veggie diet?

There's not enough research to give a precise amount. "Diet is a continuum," says Robert Ostfeld, M.D., MSc., cardiologist, and founder and director of the Cardiac Wellness Program at Montefiore Medical Center in New York. "But patients who more fully embrace a whole foods, plant-based diet have the best outcomes."

Still, research shows that eschewing meat all of the time

A NEW TWIST ON VEGETARIAN PASTA

New pastas made from legumes such as chickpeas, black beans, and lentils are packed with plant protein. It's a good way for people who don't care for beans to still reap the benefits of legumes.

Eat *THESE*

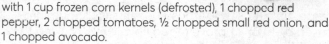

Mexican Black Bean Rotini

Combine 5 ½ cups cooked, hot, drained black bean rotini pasta with 1 cup frozen corn kernels (defrosted), 1 chopped red pepper, 2 chopped tomatoes, ½ chopped small red onion, and 1 chopped avocado.

For the dressing, combine ¼ cup fresh lime juice, ⅓ cup olive oil, ½ teaspoon salt, and ⅛ teaspoon cayenne pepper. Combine with black bean pasta mixture and top with chopped fresh cilantro.

Makes 6 servings.

Red, White and Green Rotini

Toss 4 cups cauliflower florets and 1 pint grape tomatoes in 3 tablespoons olive oil and ¼ teaspoon each salt and black pepper. Roast on a rimmed sheet pan at 425°F for 25 to 30 minutes. Add two cloves garlic, sliced, during last 5 minutes. Cook an 8-ounce package of red lentil rotini and then drain, reserving 1 cup of pasta water. Return pasta to pot. Stir in cauliflower mixture, 5 ounces of baby spinach, ½ cup grated Asiago cheese, and enough pasta water to moisten.

Makes 4 servings.

Chickpea Fusilli Formaggio

Toss 3 ½ cups cooked, drained hot pasta with ¼ cup olive oil, ¼ cup grated Parmesan cheese, and fresh parsley.

Makes 4 servings.

isn't necessary. In one recent preliminary study of more than 450,000 adults, those who followed a diet that was 70 percent plants had a 20 percent lower risk of dying from heart disease or stroke than those whose diets centered on meat and dairy.

A Harvard study that tracked more than 120,000 people for 30 years found that those who ate the most red meat tended to die younger during the study period but that swapping just one daily serving of beef for nuts could cut the risk of dying early by as much as 19 percent.

One possible reason for those benefits is that a plant-focused diet can improve blood lipid levels. Making the change from a typical American diet to a plant-based (including some meat) or vegetarian one was associated with a 10- to 15-percent decrease in total and LDL "bad" cholesterol according to a review of 27 studies in the *American Journal of Cardiology*. Shifting to a vegan diet led to even more dramatic change. A "less meat, more plants" style of eating can also help improve the quality of your life.

In addition, shifting to a plant-based diet is associated with higher levels of short-chain fatty acids in the gut. Research suggests that it lowers the risk of heart disease, inflammatory diseases, and type 2 diabetes.

A Mediterranean-style diet, based on produce, legumes, grains, and healthy oils, with small amounts of fish and meat, is connected with better brain health in older adults according to a study in the journal *Neurology*.

Those who favored fruits and vegetables along with some fish had less brain shrinkage, than those who

ate more meat. Eating no more than 3.5 ounces of meat daily may help prevent the loss of brain cells equivalent to about three or four years of aging, researchers say.

But can changing your diet after age 50 still make a difference? Absolutely, according to experts. "It's never too early or too late to embrace a healthier lifestyle," Ostfeld says. "The benefits come quickly and continue to accrue with time." In one study, women in that age group who ate a mostly plant diet were 34 percent more likely to be free of chronic diseases, like type 2 diabetes and heart disease, 15 years later than women whose diets included more meat.

HOW TO MAKE THE SWITCH:

Any step you take will help, but the more plants and fewer animal foods, the better. Try these easy tips:

1. *Up your vegetable and fruit intake.* Even if you don't actively cut back on meat at first, adding more produce will help you develop a taste for plant foods and transition to a higher-fiber diet. "I recommend including vegetables at just about every meal and snack, even breakfast," Palmer says. "Try sliced radishes on your toast or have a side of baked tomato halves."

2. *Redesign your plate.* Fill more than half of your plate with produce, grains, or beans and downsize your meat serving. Think of a stir-fry heavy on the veggies and grains with thinly sliced strips of beef rather than a big steak with a spear of broccoli. Swap in chopped mushrooms or tofu for half of the ground meat you'd normally use in meatloaf, tacos, chili, or pasta sauce. Or try veggie-based dishes like burritos.

3. *Pick the healthiest meats.* You might want to focus first on decreasing the amount of processed meat you eat —

bacon, deli meats, hot dogs, and sausage. A Harvard study linked a daily serving equal to one hot dog or two slices of bacon to an increased risk of early death from heart disease and cancer.

A group of 22 experts from 10 countries convened by the World Health Organization categorized processed meat as "carcinogenic to humans." Each 1.8 ounces of processed meat eaten daily raises the risk of colorectal cancer by 18 percent, their report says. Red meat also has been associated with heart disease and cancer risk, but the evidence is less clear. When you do eat red meat, it's best to stick to small amounts and choose lean cuts, such as pork tenderloin and top sirloin steak. And try to eat fatty fish such as salmon, which is high in inflammation-reducing omega-3 fatty acids.

4. Find your semi-veg style. Plant-based meals once every seven days in the style of Meatless Monday — a campaign that encourages people to start each week with a day of vegetarian eating — are a great way to begin. You can try replacing your meat ounce-for-ounce with a faux meat such as tempeh or tofu, Palmer says. More restrictive but also forgiving is the VB6 approach, where you eat vegan (no meat, fish, dairy, or eggs) before 6 p.m. You're free to have meat, fish, eggs, or dairy at dinner.

HAVE A GREAT VEGGIE DAY

So you're sold on the idea of shifting to a more vegetarian diet. If only you knew what to eat. Here's a day's worth of completely plant-based meals to mix into your normal routine, putting you on the road to becoming a flexitarian.

BREAKFAST: Avocado Toast
2 slices whole-grain bread, mashed avocado, red-pepper flakes, salt, coffee with coconut-milk creamer.

LUNCH: Quinoa Tabbouleh with Chickpeas
Cooked quinoa, chopped tomatoes, chopped cucumber, chopped parsley, olive oil, lemon juice, black olives, chickpeas.

AFTERNOON SNACK: Fruit-and-Nuts Bar
Choose a bar that has 200 or fewer calories. Make sure real foods are high on the ingredient list, such as oats, raisins, blueberries, nuts, dates, and dried cranberries. Soy protein or chicory root listed as the first ingredient means that the manufacturer boosted protein and fiber with less wholesome ingredients.

DINNER: Black-Bean Tacos
Corn tortillas, black beans, roasted cauliflower, jarred corn salsa, pico de gallo, cumin, salad greens.

SNACK: Frozen Banana "Ice Cream"
Blend a frozen banana with a touch of almond milk until it resembles soft serve, topped with chopped walnuts.

4 FOODS THAT HELP KEEP YOU YOUNG

Would you rather add years to your life or life to your years? Smart food choices may help you do *both*.

Diet appears to play a role in free-radical damage (which alters cells' functioning), inflammation, and gut bacteria. Diet also affects the length of telomeres — protective caps at the end of chromosomes. These factors can have an impact on conditions like heart disease, type 2 diabetes, stroke, hypertension, respiratory disorders, cognitive decline, and infection.

"We're trying to target the biology of aging to delay the onset of age-related diseases and extend the number of healthy, active, productive years," says Nathan LeBrasseur, Ph.D., director of the Healthy Aging and Independent Living Program at the Mayo Clinic. "Diet can play a major role in that." Though following an overall healthy diet is most important, research suggests that incorporating certain foods into your diet may give you an extra boost. Here, four foods to consider:

1. Beans. Beans are rich in protein, fiber, vitamins, minerals, and plant polyphenols that have protective benefits, especially for your heart. A large research review in the *American Journal of Clinical Nutrition* found that eating four half-cup servings of beans, peas, lentils, or tofu per week was linked to a 14-percent decrease in the risk of dying from ischemic heart disease (when the arteries of the heart become blocked). Beans are a good source of soluble fiber too, which helps lower levels of LDL ("bad") cholesterol and triglycerides.

2. Hot peppers. If you can tolerate them, chilies are good for your heart and waistline. A large study published in 2017 in the journal *PLOS ONE*, found that people who ate hot red chili peppers regularly were 13 percent less likely to die from any cause over a 19-year period compared with those who didn't. Capsaicin, which gives peppers their heat, may also help improve blood flow, boost metabolism, and protect against bacteria that have been linked with inflammation and diseases.

"Inflammation is the nail in the coffin of conditions like heart disease, rheumatoid arthritis, inflammatory bowel disease, type 2 diabetes, cancer, and more," says Carin Kreutzer, Ed.D., R.D., an assistant instructional professor of nutrition at the University of Southern California Leonard Davis School of Gerontology. "Many plant foods have phytochemicals that reduce the inflammatory response at the cellular level."

In addition to green and red chilies, cayenne, jalapeño, and tabasco peppers all contain high levels of capsaicin. Sweeter peppers have less of that compound.

3. Nuts. Research suggests that nuts may be tiny packages of healthy goodness. Take, for example, a study in *The New England Journal of Medicine* that followed almost 120,000 men and women for 30 years. Study volunteers who ate at least an ounce of nuts (about 23 almonds, 18 cashews, 12 macadamia nuts, or 14 walnut halves) daily had a 20-percent-lower risk of dying from several conditions— especially cancer, heart disease, and respiratory problems — during the study period. Even those who downed nuts two to four times per week had a 13-percent-lower risk of dying.

Nuts are high in monounsaturated fat, which helps lower LDL (bad) cholesterol. Studies have also shown that nuts' antioxidants may keep blood vessels supple (hardened arteries are a sign of heart disease) and improve your body's use of insulin. Nuts have about 160 to 200 calories per ounce, but in the study above, frequent nut eaters weighed less than those who abstained.

4. Fish. Fatty fish is high in inflammation-fighting omega-3 fatty acids, which may help protect the heart and brain. Some research has shown a significant 33-percent drop in the risk of sudden heart attack death in people who ate two or more servings per week. Some interesting preliminary research shows that people with cognitive impairments who supplemented with EPA and DHA — omega-3 fatty acids found in certain types of fish — had less telomere shortening over time.

Studies of supplements have had mixed results, and experts advise getting your dose with fish. Try for 8 ounces per week of sustainably farmed or wild-caught, low-mercury fish, such as Atlantic mackerel, Pacific sardines, freshwater (farmed) coho salmon and wild-caught salmon, and sablefish (black cod) from Alaska.

Lentil and Spinach Soup

2 tbsp olive oil

1 large onion, chopped

2 cloves garlic, minced

2 cups uncooked lentils

4 cups low-sodium vegetable broth

4 cups water

1 sprig (2–3 inches) fresh rosemary

1 (7-oz) package baby spinach, roughly chopped

2 large tomatoes, chopped

½ tsp black pepper

Heat oil in large pot over medium heat. Add onion and garlic; cook until onion is soft, about 5 minutes, stirring often. Add lentils, broth, water, and rosemary and bring to a boil. Reduce heat and simmer uncovered until lentils are tender, about 20 minutes. Add spinach and tomatoes and simmer for 10 minutes. Remove rosemary sprig. Stir in pepper. Serve or refrigerate. (Bring refrigerated soup to a boil before serving.)

Makes about 10 cups

NUTRITION AT A GLANCE
Calories 170, Fat 3.5 g, Saturated fat 0,
Protein 9 g, Fiber 7 g, Sodium 80 mg

---

4 FOODS THAT CAN COST YOU YEARS

Fill your plate with the four following kinds of foods and you may hike your risk of heart disease, cancer, and a variety of other serious illnesses. Avoid or limit:

1. *Charred meat.* Studies have found that grilled or well-done meat creates compounds that have been linked to an increased risk of colon, pancreatic, stomach, and possibly other cancers.

2. *Processed meats.* Though red meat in general has been associated with an increased risk of colon cancer, salami, pepperoni, ham, and other cured meats may predispose you to esophageal, kidney, stomach, and prostate cancer.

3. *Refined carbohydrates.* Diets that are high in added sugars (candy, some cereals, pastries, sodas) and carbohydrates that have been stripped of many of their important nutrients (these are carbs such as white flour and white rice) may shorten telomeres and hike the risk of type 2 diabetes, obesity, heart disease, and stroke, especially in those who are overweight.

4. *Prepackaged meals.* They may be convenient, but they are often extremely high in sodium. That has been linked to a higher risk of hypertension, cardiovascular disease, and kidney disease.

QUIET MEALS, HEALTHIER CHOICES

You may want to turn down the volume at dinnertime. Families that ate as a vacuum cleaner roared nearby consumed 34 percent more cookies than those that dined in a more peaceful setting according to a University of Illinois study.

WHEN YOU EAT CAN IMPACT YOUR HEALTH

A scientific statement from the American Heart Association released in 2017 suggests that it's not just *what* you eat, it's *when* you eat it.

Here are three "timing" habits that show promise in helping to prevent heart disease and related conditions, such as type 2 diabetes and obesity.

1. Intermittent fasting. Studies suggest severely limiting your calorie intake one or two days per week may help with weight loss and reduce triglycerides, blood pressure, and insulin resistance.

"We've known for a long time that calorie restriction can delay the onset of age-related conditions and diseases. Now we have newer data on intermittent fasting and time-restricted feeding that's dramatic and promising," says Mayo Clinic's Nathan LeBrasseur, Ph.D.

2. Meal timing. Some studies suggest that people who consume most of their calories late in the day have a higher risk of obesity and heart disease. Research published in the *American Journal of Clinical Nutrition* found that consuming 50 percent of daily calories at lunch and 20 percent at dinner led to about a 33-percent-greater weight loss than eating 50 percent at dinner.

Similarly, restricting calories to a 10- to 12-hour period may be beneficial for dropping pounds.

3. Eating breakfast. It's associated with a better blood glucose and insulin balance, which may lower type 2 diabetes and obesity risks.

CHAPTER FOUR

DRINK

Sip *THIS*
to shield yourself from disease

Matcha tea is a green tea made with the whole leaf. Matcha tea has more EGCG, an antioxidant that may help protect against cancer and heart disease, than other green teas do. Matcha tea also contains L-theanine, a compound that may help you feel focused and alert. Snack bars, ice cream, and other foods made with matcha are less likely to have the same benefits as a cup of matcha tea, probably because the foods contain less matcha.

IN THIS CHAPTER:

JUICY CLAIMS

Cleanse makers promise health and well-being in a bottle. Should you believe them?

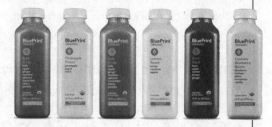

BOTTOMS UP: *BluePrint* boasts that its $195 three-day cleanses eliminate toxins and cleanse the blood. We found nothing that proves such powers.

Almost 20 percent of adults who want to lose or maintain weight have tried a "cleanse."

Adults ages 18 to 34 are the biggest cleanse users, with men edging out women according to market research firm Mintel. And it costs bottled juice cleanse buyers more than $200 million each year. On a cleanse, you replace solid food with fruit and vegetable juices (and sometimes nut milks) for one day to a week or longer. Although weight loss is one reason people try cleanses, certain manufacturers say their products will "reset your body," "eliminate toxins," and more. And cleanses come complete with healthy-sounding names such as *Glow* and *Purify*.

That's heady stuff for any juice. To find out whether they live up to the hype, in September 2015 Consumer Reports ordered a three-day program from several brands including *BluePrint's® Renovation Cleanse, Suja's Original Fresh Start™*, and *Pressed Juicery's Cleanse 1*. Costs range from $129 to nearly $200 per cleanse. After evaluating ingredients, reviewing medical research, and talking to experts, we put those health claims into perspective.

THE CLAIM: *Removes toxins*

THE REALITY: Our bodies make toxins — like urea (a compound produced when we digest protein) and lactic acid (which our muscles make during strenuous exercise). "But we don't need help removing them," says nephrologist Orlando Gutierrez, M.D., associate professor of medicine at the University of Alabama at Birmingham. "The kidneys and liver are the body's natural detoxers."

THE CLAIM: *Rests your digestive system*

THE REALITY: "Unless you have a condition such as inflammatory bowel disease or Crohn's disease, it's not necessary to rest your digestive system," says Arthur

What you should eat vs. what's in a juice cleanse

On average, these cleanses are too high in carbohydrates — especially sugars — and too low in fiber and protein.

Recommended daily distribution of calories

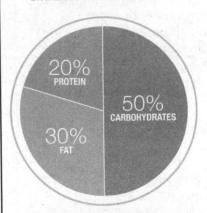

20% PROTEIN

50% CARBOHYDRATES

30% FAT

Beginner cleanse average daily distribution of calories

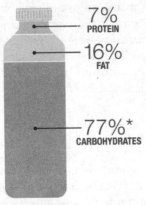

7% PROTEIN

16% FAT

77%* CARBOHYDRATES

Fiber: 28 grams for a 2,000 calorie-per-day diet

Fiber: 14 grams

*Approximately 80 percent of total carbohydrates are primarily from naturally occuring sugars.

Heller, M.D., a gastroenterologist at New York-Presbyterian Hospital/ Weill Cornell Medical Center. In fact, many cleanses are very low in fiber, a component that helps your digestive system run smoothly.

THE CLAIM: *Takes off weight*

THE REALITY: None of the cleanses we looked at promised you'd drop pounds, but that's an important reason many people try one, says Consumer Reports dietitian, Amy Keating, R.D. And you probably will lose weight because the three-day programs range from just 735 to 1,520 calories per day. But the majority of that will be water weight, which will probably come back if you return to eating your typical diet.

THE CLAIM: *Reduces your dependence on unhealthy, processed foods*

THE REALITY: Cleanses can make you temporarily feel healthier, "not because they contain something miraculous, but because if you follow the program, you'll be eliminating not-so-good-for-you foods from your diet for that stretch of time," Keating says. If you're healthy and aren't pregnant or breastfeeding, doing one of the cleanses for up to three days probably won't harm you. But longer isn't wise because you won't get the nutrients your body needs.

DON'T sip the juice *when you can eat the whole fruit*

Juice lacks the dietary fiber found in whole fruit, which may help reduce heart disease risk, control weight, and aid digestion.

Juice also has more calories per serving than whole fruit — 112 calories in an 8-ounce serving of 100-percent orange juice, for example, compared with 65 calories in a medium-sized orange.

COFFEE PERKS

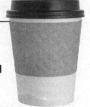

Coffee in moderation can be a very good thing. But too much can be a bad thing. What you need to know.

The headlines about coffee's impact on your health seem to change as quickly as the time it takes to drink a cup.

We still don't know everything about caffeine. Caffeine is speedily and completely absorbed through the intestines, so you can get that eye-opening pop in as little as 10 minutes. Once in the brain, it targets and blocks a cascade of neu- rotransmitter signals that would normally make you sleepy.

But caffeine can also have other effects on your body, both positive and negative. Though more research is needed, studies have indicated that caffeine could both precipitate and alleviate headache, boost athletic performance and memory, protect against type 2 diabetes, worsen incontinence, prevent constipation, and exacerbate menopausal hot flashes.

And that leaves us with the question: *Should you savor every drop — or try to cut down?* Here's what we know right now.

1. *Coffee may make you happier.* Coffee is not just a pick-me-up — it also has been linked to a lower risk of depression. In a study led by the Harvard School of Public Health, people who drank four or more cups of caffeinated coffee per day were 20 percent less likely to develop depression than nondrinkers.

2. *It may protect you from disease and even lengthen your life.* Researchers found that people ages 50 to 71 who drank at least one cup of coffee per day lowered their risk of

dying from diabetes, heart disease, or other health problems when followed for more than a decade.

That may be due to beneficial compounds such as antioxidants — which might ward off disease — and not caffeine. For most Americans who drink coffee, it provides more antioxidants than any other food according to Joe Vinson, Ph.D., a chemistry professor at the University of Scranton. Decaf drinkers had the same results.

THE CAFFEINE COUNT

Caffeine can be found in a number of foods and beverages — even where you wouldn't expect it — sometimes in doses higher than in coffee. Consuming too many of those foods and drinks can quickly put you over the 400 mg daily limit set by the Department of Agriculture's Dietary Guidelines for Americans.

200 mg
per 1.9 ounces
5-hour ENERGY®
Regular Strength

195 mg
per 12 ounces
Starbucks
Dark Roast,
Tall

160 mg
per 16 ounces
Hiball Sparkling
Energy Water

150 mg
per 2 tablespoons
STEEM
Caffeinated
Peanut Butter

125 mg
per 1/2 cup
Bang!!
Caffeinated
Ice Cream

100 mg
per 1 mint
FOOSH®
Energy Mints

87 mg
per 16.9
ounces
Unsweet
Lemon
Honest Tea

80 mg
per 8.4
ounces
Red Bull

50 mg
per 1 ounce
Extreme Sport
Beans®

49 mg
per 1 bar
CLIF BAR®
Cool Mint
Chocolate®

46 mg
per 12
ounces
Diet Coke®

30 mg
per 6 ounces
Dannon Coffee
Yogurt

20 mg
per 1.45
ounces
Hershey's
Special Dark
Chocolate

3. _It's not for everyone._ More than 500 mg of caffeine — or about four to five cups of brewed coffee — per day can cause side effects including insomnia, irritability, and restlessness. Caffeine stimulates the central nervous system, heart, and muscles. So if you have an anxiety disorder, irritable bowel syndrome, or heart disease, or if you take certain medications, watch your consumption or opt for decaf. And if you have acid reflux, you might want to skip coffee altogether because the acidity could exacerbate it.

4. _Be mindful of drinking coffee with other caffeinated drinks or foods._ Pairing a cup of java with caffeinated versions of yogurt and peanut butter at breakfast may sound like a boon, but it may be too much caffeine for you to handle at once. There's a difference between getting 400 mg of caffeine over the course of a day and consuming that amount or more in one sitting, notes Neal Benowitz, M.D., professor of medicine at the University of California, San Francisco. "With drugs that affect mood or behavior such as caffeine, the faster the rise in the drug level in the body, the more intense the response," Benowitz says. To prevent a big punch, be mindful of your own tolerance. If you start to feel nervous or jittery, you've probably had too much.

QUESTION: *GOT MILK?*
ANSWER: *YES!*

There are more kinds of milk out there than ever — soy, almond, coconut. But just as dizzying is the array of choices for plain old cow's milk. Our milk primer can help.

Q. Should I opt for organic milk?

A. *If you can afford the extra $1 or so per half gallon, yes.* The USDA rules require organic dairy farms to use 100-percent organic feed, no growth hormones, and no antibiotics. Buying organic also supports healthy agricultural practices. Organic milk from grassfed cows costs a little more but some studies show it has slightly more conjugated linoleic acid (CLA) and other healthy fatty acids.

Q. Is omega-3-fortified milk a good choice?

A. *It has 32 to 50 milligrams of omega-3s per glass —* a fraction of the 500 milligrams per day suggested for heart health. Plus the omegas are added in the form of flavorless fish oil or algae oil, so it's like swallowing a mini-supplement with your milk. That's not ideal. Research suggests that omega-3 supplements may not be as effective as the real thing: It's better to have two servings of fatty fish per week.

Q. What makes "creamy" skim milks like *Skim Plus®* so creamy?

A. *Manufacturers can make "fat-free" cream by adding milk solids or filtering to remove water and some of the milk sugar.* Eight ounces have about 40 more calories, 3 extra protein grams, and 100 milligrams more calcium than regular skim milk, but the same amount of fat.

Q. Is milk made from nuts, such as almond and cashew milk, healthful?

A. *It can be.* The biggest difference between nut-based milk and dairy milk is that the nut-based doesn't naturally contain the high amount of calcium found in dairy milk. So if you want calcium too, look for brands fortified with calcium. The other big difference is the protein content: about 8 grams per one-cup serving of dairy milk vs. just 1 gram in a serving of almond milk and 0 grams in cashew milk. Nut milk might contain some vitamins and other nutrients not found in regular milk, such as fiber and vitamin E.

Q. *Nonfat, 1 percent, 2 percent — what's the difference?*

A. *More than you think. Compare eight ounces of each type of cow's milk:*

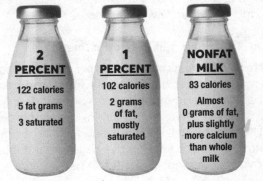

2 PERCENT

122 calories

5 fat grams

3 saturated

1 PERCENT

102 calories

2 grams of fat, mostly saturated

NONFAT MILK

83 calories

Almost 0 grams of fat, plus slightly more calcium than whole milk

4 TIPS TO MAKE HEALTHY SMOOTHIES

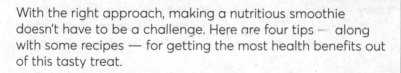

Healthy smoothies. Those words often go hand in hand, but many smoothies aren't healthy at all. In fact, they often have more calories and sugars than a serving of ice cream.

With the right approach, making a nutritious smoothie doesn't have to be a challenge. Here are four tips — along with some recipes — for getting the most health benefits out of this tasty treat.

1. *Blend it yourself.* Store-bought and pre-bottled smoothies may be convenient, but they can be packed with excess calories, fat, and sugars. For example, a small *Jamba Juice "Strawberry Surf Rider™"* has 320 calories and a whopping 70 grams (about 17 teaspoons) of sugars. Some of those grams come from the natural sugars in the peaches and strawberries of course, but it's also sweetened with a lemonade and sherbet blend, which are full of added sugars. Health authorities recommend that 10 percent or less of your daily calories come from added sugars. So if you're on an 1,800-calorie-per-day diet, you should be getting no more than 45 grams.

You might also be surprised to find that sodium levels in store-bought smoothies can be high. Order a small serving of *"The Shredder — Strawberry™"* at *Smoothie King*, and you'll get 300 milligrams (along with 340 calories). That's quite a bit of sodium, considering most people are only supposed to have 2,300 mg per day.

2. Load up on the veggies. Many of us have trouble incorporating a variety of vegetables into our daily diet, but if you sneak them into smoothies, it can help up your intake. If you use a blender, as compared to some juicers, you'll get all of the vegetable's fiber, which helps you feel full. Sweeter

---

Sip *THESE*

Many smoothies are refreshing and delicious, but it's not so easy to find one that's also nutritious. Made with whole fruit and vegetables, each of these four drinks is a tasty way to sneak in some of the recommended intake of "five a day." They're also packed with protein and fiber, so they're perfect for a healthy breakfast or snack.

Lean green dream. Toss some kale into your smoothie, and you'll get the nutritious boost without any bitter flavor.

In a blender, add 1 banana frozen then thawed for 15 to 20 minutes, 2 cups chopped kale, ½ cup almond milk, and 1 tablespoon honey. Blend until smooth. Makes 1 serving.

Per serving: 260 calories, 3 g fat, 125 mg sodium, 6 g fiber, 35 g sugars, 8 g protein.

Chocoholic's delight. Sure, it's packed with healthy protein and potassium, but the taste of this morning milkshake is pure chocolate goodness.

In a blender, add 1 medium banana frozen then thawed for 15 to 20 minutes, 4 ounces silken tofu, ½ cup chocolate almond milk, 1 tablespoon unsweetened cocoa powder, ½ teaspoon cinnamon. Blend until smooth. Makes 1 serving.

Per serving: 230 calories, 5 g fat, 80 mg sodium, 6 g fiber, 25 g sugars, 8 g protein

veggies like beets and carrots are good choices, but you can mask the bitter taste of highly nutritious dark leafy greens, such as kale and spinach, by combining them with fruit in your mix. Try tossing a handful of kale or spinach into any smoothie recipe.

Fruit-and-fiber frappé. You could eat your yogurt, then a bowl of fruit, then your oatmeal, with a glass of juice on the side — or throw it all in a blender for a three-course breakfast in a glass.

In a blender, add ¼ cup oats and blend until powdery. Add 1 ½ cups frozen mixed berries, ½ cup nonfat plain Greek yogurt, ¼ cup orange juice, 1 tablespoon maple syrup, and 1 teaspoon orange zest. Blend until smooth. Makes 1 serving.

Per serving: 320 calories, 2.5 g fat, 45 mg sodium, 8 g fiber, 39 g sugars, 17 g protein

Tropical temptation. It's like having a piña colada — no airfare to the islands required. Tiny umbrella optional.

In a blender, add 1 cup frozen tropical fruit mix (pineapple, mango, and papaya), 1 6-ounce container nonfat plain Greek yogurt, ½ cup unsweetened coconut almond milk, 2 teaspoons sugar. Blend until smooth. Garnish with fresh fruit if desired. Makes 1 serving.

Per serving: 240 calories, 2.5 g fat, 130 mg sodium, 3 g fiber, 32 g sugars, 19 g protein

3. Skip the extras. Bee pollen, creatine, conjugated linoleic acid (CLA), green tea powder, guarana, vitamin C — these are just a few of the extras found in so-called healthy smoothies available at smoothie shops, gyms, and supermarkets. You'll often see some kind of claim attached to these extras — more energy, muscle builder, immune system booster, burn fat faster, to name a few. The problem isn't just that these claims have little, if any, good evidence behind them, but some of the ingredients can be harmful if consumed in excess. For example, guarana naturally contains caffeine. Up to 400 mg of caffeine — the amount in two to four 8-ounce cups of coffee — per day can be part of a healthy diet for most adults, but chances are you won't know how much caffeine guarana adds to your smoothie.

What about extra vitamins and minerals? You can skip those too. The vast majority of people can meet their nutrient needs with food alone.

When you start adding high doses of vitamins and minerals to the amount you get from foods, you risk overdoing it, and that can have negative effects. *Naked* brand's *"Power-C Machine"* smoothie, for example, packs 1,900 percent of the daily vitamin C recommended in one 15-ounce serving. According to the National Institutes of Health, too much vitamin C can cause abdominal cramps, diarrhea, nausea, and other intestinal problems.

4. Add creaminess the healthy way. Almond and soy milks, avocados, low-fat yogurts, and nut butters can give you that smooth texture and add some healthy fats to your smoothies. Toss in some flax or chia seeds, which are not only a good source of heart-healthy omega-3 fatty acids but also contain decent amounts of fiber, protein, and vitamins. Frozen fruit also adds that satisfying thickness.

GO AHEAD AND WINE

Research shows that pouring yourself a glass now and then can be beneficial to your health — but moderation is key.

If you have seen the headlines touting the health benefits of wine — and you're among the 31 percent of drinkers who prefer a glass of wine to other alcoholic beverages — you've probably been thrilled to watch a former vice morph into a virtue. But before you get too carried away celebrating, there are a few facts you should know about how alcohol consumption really affects your health.

THE BENEFITS
"The association between moderate alcohol intake and lower risk of myocardial infarction (heart attack) has been studied in well-designed observational studies for nearly 50 years," says Kenneth Mukamal, M.D., M.P.H., a professor of medicine at Harvard Medical School.

THE RISKS
Alcohol has been linked to a small increased risk of cancer. A study published in the *British Medical Journal (BMJ)* found that moderate drinkers had a 2 to 6 percent higher risk than nondrinkers.

But the association between moderate alcohol intake and the risk of breast cancer was stronger. Women who drank the amount of alcohol in one-third to one glass of wine per day had a 13-percent-increased risk of cancer, mostly driven by breast cancer.

Once drinking goes beyond the small amounts defined as moderate, the risks quickly start to outweigh any potential cardiovascular benefits. Higher levels of alcohol intake are linked to increases in heart disease, high blood pressure, heart attack, and stroke, as well as various types of cancer.

No matter which studies you look at, any purported benefits associated with drinking are related specifically to "moderate" consumption: one drink per day for women and up to two for men. Men are allowed more to account for their generally larger size and differences in the way they metabolize alcohol. For wine, one drink is 5 ounces. See what that looks like in five glasses, below.

If you stick to those amounts, the evidence is pretty clear that alcohol can boost your heart health.

WHAT 5 OUNCES LOOKS LIKE

When health experts say a glass of wine is good for your health, they're talking about a 5-ounce serving. Depending on the size and shape of the glass you choose, that can look very different.

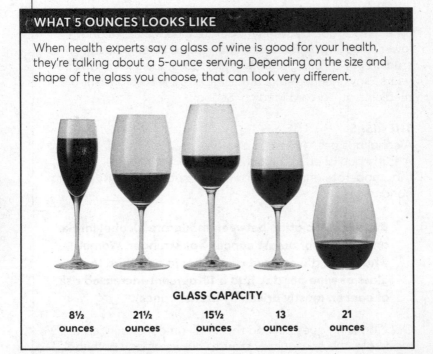

GLASS CAPACITY

| 8½ ounces | 21½ ounces | 15½ ounces | 13 ounces | 21 ounces |

THE UNKNOWNS

The data on alcohol is fairly consistent, but most of the studies don't prove cause and effect. Many are observational — that is, they look at what people do in their lives rather than randomly assign people to drink or abstain from alcohol, then follow them to see the effects on their health. The latter type of study would be ideal, but creating a placebo for alcohol to give to a control group is tricky. And attempting to separate large groups of subjects and randomly instruct them to drink or not drink for several years has proven to be almost impossible.

Without that clinical evidence, some experts are reluctant to recommend moderate drinking as a health tactic.

"The observational data is good, but what limited experimental evidence we have shows no benefit to moderate drinking," says Michael Criqui, M.D., M.P.H., a professor in the division of preventive medicine at the University of California, San Diego. Therefore, the American Heart Association and other health organizations advise that if you do drink alcohol, do so in moderation. And if you don't, you shouldn't start.

SHOULD YOU DRINK WINE?

As long as you raise just one glass (or two if you're a guy), the health risks are pretty small. But rather than kid yourself that you're doing something super-healthy, just sip and enjoy — in moderation.

CHOOSE THE HEALTHIEST TEA

Lower your body mass index and improve your health, simply by sipping tea.

As the most sipped beverage worldwide after water, tea is far from a new trend. However, with several varieties available and research linking tea with many health benefits, you may be wondering which type should be your, well, cup of tea. We'll make it easy: All of them!

> **Whether it's black, green, oolong, or white, tea offers a no-calorie way to up your intake of disease-fighting plant compounds.**

"In the U.S., tea drinkers have the highest flavonoid intake," says Jeffrey Blumberg, Ph.D., professor of nutrition at Tufts University, referring to the antioxidants responsible for many of tea's health benefits. "We're talking about a flavorful, aromatic, healthful beverage," Blumberg adds.

Tea has antioxidants and other compounds that may protect against cancer, heart disease, osteoporosis, and memory decline. Researchers at Penn State University found that people who drank multiple cups of hot tea each day had a body mass index 3 points lower, on average, than non-tea drinkers. To get the most antioxidants, let the tea steep for 3 minutes.

Remember that adding milk to your tea could block the absorption of some of the antioxidants.

HOW MUCH SHOULD YOU DRINK?
There's no standard recommendation — as with other plant

foods. More is generally a good thing, within reason. Some experts recommend having 2 to 3 cups per day. Just be sure to balance your tea intake with your tolerance for caffeine (or favor decaffeinated varieties).

TYPES OF TEA AND THEIR HEALTH BENEFITS

BLACK

It may help strengthen your skeleton. Post-menopausal women who regularly drank black tea had higher bone mineral density in the lumbar spine and hip according to a Japanese study that tracked 498 women over five years. Just skip the splash of milk, at least some of the time — its proteins can bind with some of the beneficial compounds in black tea, reducing your body's ability to absorb them, researchers say.

GREEN

Green tea gets a lot of attention for being a good source of the plant compound epigallocatechin gallate (EGCG), found in studies to decrease LDL (bad) cholesterol. EGCG may also counter inflammation in the body.

Squeezing a slice of lemon into green tea may help its beneficial compounds survive digestion according to research from Purdue University.

WHITE

White teas contain the most catechins, a type of flavonoid that may help keep blood vessels open and help the body break down fat.

CHAPTER FIVE

PROTECT

Don't Eat *THIS*
if you want to avoid
excess salt

Aunt Jemima® Original *Pancake and Waffle Mix* has MORE sodium per serving than *Wise Golden Original Potato Chips* and *Planters Salted Peanuts* combined! Sodium lurks in places you might not suspect. Read the labels of convenience foods carefully. And when preparing meals, don't salt food while cooking. The salty taste evaporates somewhat during cooking, but when you sprinkle salt onto already cooked foods, it comes through clearly.

IN THIS CHAPTER:

HOW TO LOSE WEIGHT AND KEEP IT OFF

Sure, losing weight to look better is a good incentive. But losing weight, if you need to, and maintaining a healthy weight are also keys to protecting good, long-term health.

Many people call a truce with the battle of the bulge at a certain age, and that's not necessarily a bad thing.

When you're over 60, being a little overweight may be beneficial, because being underweight increases the risk of malnutrition, osteoporosis, and falls.

But you don't want to be carrying too much excess weight. "If you're very overweight or obese, you're more likely to develop chronic diseases earlier in life," says Steven Heymsfield, M.D., a professor at the Pennington Biomedical Research Center at Louisiana State University.

Weight gain with age is common. "Your metabolism gradually slows down," Heymsfield says. Sarcopenia, a decrease in muscle tissue that occurs with age, is a likely cause — but not the only one. "People generally become less active as they get older, even more so if they have orthopedic or other painful health issues," he says. "When you're not burning as many calories but still eating the same amount, you gradually gain weight."

Prescription medications may also play a role. Certain classes of antidepressants, antipsychotics, and corticosteroids can lead to substantial weight gain.

You probably don't have to lose as much weight as you think you do to improve your health.

Simply maintaining a healthy weight—or dropping just a few pounds if necessary—can be worthwhile. "Losing just 5 to 8 percent of your weight (about 11 to 17 pounds for a 220-pound person) improves your health and how well you function," Heymsfield says. The effect can be considerable:

- If you have high blood pressure, losing 9 pounds can reduce systolic blood pressure by 4.5 points and diastolic by 3 points according to a 2014 review by the Cochrane Collaboration.

- A study published in *The New England Journal of Medicine* found that people who lost 7 percent of their weight had a 58-percent-lower risk of developing type 2 diabetes.

- A 2016 study in *Cell Metabolism*, which looked at the effects of weight loss on 40 obese people, found that those who dropped 5 percent of their body weight substantially cut their risk for type 2 diabetes and heart disease.

- Being overweight may increase the risk of cancers such as breast, colon, and endometrial, as well as osteoarthritis, heart disease, type 2 diabetes, and eye diseases such as age-related cataracts.

- Research from the Harvard Medical School found that women with high levels of abdominal fat tend to have lower bone mineral density.

"Changing a diet has to be something you can stick with long term because if you return to the way you were eating before, you'll likely gain back the weight," says Denise K. Houston, R.D., Ph.D., an associate professor of gerontology and geriatric medicine at the Wake Forest School of Medicine.

8 HEALTHY EATING TIPS FOR WEIGHT LOSS

1. *Change your perspective.* Instead of thinking of yourself as someone who is dieting, consider yourself a "weight manager," advises Andrea Spivack, R.D., with the Stunkard Weight Management Program at the University of Pennsylvania.

2. *Be ready for challenges.* Use a calendar to mark social events for the month ahead. This will give you perspective on how many situations may test your willpower. Strive to stay on track the rest of the time. Note on the calendar when you plan to exercise.

3. *Cook at home more often.* Cooking at home can help you control your weight and improve your health. Home-cooked meals may help because they're usually lower in calories, fat, and sodium, and contain more nutrient-and fiber-rich produce than restaurant fare, fast food, and takeout meals. Finding time to cook at home can be a challenge. To make it a little easier, see the six delicious, fast, filling dishes you can make at home starting on page 45.

4. *Put your fork down between each bite.* This gives your brain more time to receive the message that you're full. Another recent study found that people reported less hunger after eating slowly.

5. *Avoid processed foods.* Think freshness and variety. Try to cut down on packaged foods with lots of ingredients you would not normally find in a kitchen cupboard and sound like they are from the lab.

6. *Steer clear of high-protein, low-carb diets.* Diets like the *Zone, Paleo, Atkins,* and more claim that you'll lose weight, feel peppier, and reduce your risk of heart disease. Sure, these diets can help you lose weight — but only by lowering calories. It doesn't matter where the calories come from. Many of these plans recommend cutting back on carbs or eliminating carbs. Get less than 50 grams of carbs per day (the amount in two apples) and in three or four days your body will start to tap muscles for fuel. This can cause serious health consequences and problems with brain function.

7. *Reconsider grazing.* Keeping your nibbling to a smaller chunk of the day could aid weight loss. In one study, overweight subjects grazed 15 hours or more on most days. But when they contained their grazing time to 10 to 11 hours a day, they lost an average of 7 pounds in 16 weeks.

8. *Be kind to yourself.* You're seeking improvement, not perfection.

9 MEALS TO HELP YOU LOSE WEIGHT

Mix and match these meals to eat healthy all week.

This plan — 1,500 calories per day for women, 1,650 for men — will help you lose weight while still getting the nutrients you need. The dishes are listed by meal type, but you can mix and match. The breakfasts have fewer calories than the lunches and dinners. If you opt to have more than one breakfast as a meal per day, increase the portion size slightly and add a piece of fruit. Women should add one snack and one treat per day; men should have two snacks and one treat.

BREAKFAST *Pick one (350 calories each)*

TOMATO-BASIL OMELET

> 2 eggs
> 1 tbsp water
> ⅛ tsp each salt and black pepper
> 2 tomato slices cut in half
> 1 oz fresh mozzarella
> Chopped fresh basil
> Orange segments
> Chopped mint

Whisk eggs with water, salt, and pepper, and pour into a heated nonstick skillet. Swirl to cover the bottom; cook until almost firm. Add tomato, mozzarella, and basil to one side of the eggs. Fold over to create an omelet. Cook until center is warmed through, about 3 minutes. Serve with orange segments and chopped mint.

NUTTY BLUEBERRY SWEET-POTATO TOAST

Medium sweet potato, cut in half lengthwise into ¼-inch slices
2 tsp peanut or almond butter
⅓ cup blueberries
Cinnamon

Toast 2 sweet-potato slices in a toaster until soft, about two to three cycles. Spread peanut or almond butter on each slice, then top each with blueberries. Sprinkle with cinnamon to taste.

VANILLA-ORANGE FRENCH TOAST WITH HONEYED RICOTTA

1 egg
2 tbsp nonfat milk
½ tsp vanilla extract
1 tsp orange zest
Dash of cinnamon
2 slices whole-wheat bread
1½ tsp butter

Topping

¼ cup part-skim ricotta cheese
1 tsp honey
1 tsp orange zest
¾ cup berries

Whisk egg with nonfat milk, vanilla extract, orange zest, and cinnamon. Soak bread in the egg mixture, flipping to coat each side. Melt butter in skillet. Place soaked bread in skillet and cook until browned on each side, about 2 to 3 minutes. Top with a mixture of the ricotta, honey, and orange zest. Serve with berries.

ARUGULA, ORANGE, AND CHICKPEA SALAD

2 cups arugula

¾ cup chickpeas

¼ cup cooked bulgur wheat

¼ cup orange segments cut into chunks

1 tbsp sunflower seeds

2 tbsp goat cheese

Dressing

1 tsp olive oil

1 tsp lemon juice

½ tsp honey

⅛ tsp garlic powder

Toss salad ingredients together. Whisk ingredients for dressing and toss with salad.

ALMOND BUTTER AND FRUIT WRAP

1 whole-wheat tortilla

1½ tbsp almond butter

½ banana, sliced

⅓ cup sliced strawberries

Topping

4 oz plain 2% Greek yogurt

1 tsp honey

Cinnamon

Spread tortilla with almond butter and top with banana and strawberries. Roll up. Serve with yogurt mixed with honey and cinnamon for dipping.

PICNIC LUNCH

1 hard-boiled egg
¾ cup grapes
7 woven whole-wheat crackers
2 tbsp hummus
½ oz cheddar cheese

Cucumber-tomato salad

½ cucumber, sliced
2 tomato slices, quartered

Dressing

2 tsp red-wine vinegar and 1 tsp olive oil

Serve egg with grapes, crackers, hummus, cheese, and
the cucumber-tomato salad dressed with the vinegar
and olive oil.

DINNER   *Pick one (425 calories each)*

CUMIN CHICKEN WITH KALE AND BAKED FRIES

4-oz skinless chicken breast
¼ tsp each salt and ground cumin
½ tsp olive oil

Vegetables

Medium russet potato cut into ¼ -inch strips
tossed with 1 tsp olive oil
2 cups roughly chopped kale and ½ tsp olive oil
1 tsp lemon juice
⅛ tsp each chili powder, cumin, and salt

Rub chicken breast with salt, cumin, and olive oil. Place on a
large foil-lined baking sheet. Add cut potato. Bake at 425°F
for 10 minutes. Flip fries and cook about 15 minutes more, until
chicken is cooked through. Meanwhile, sauté kale in olive oil
over medium-high heat until tender, about 5 minutes. Stir in
lemon juice, chili powder, cumin, and salt.

WALNUT-CRUSTED SALMON WITH VEGETABLES

4-oz salmon fillet
⅛ tsp each salt and black pepper
1 tsp lemon juice
1 tbsp crushed walnuts mixed with 1 tsp chopped parsley

Vegetables

1 cup broccoli
1 cup baby potatoes
2 tsp olive oil
½ tsp honey
⅛ tsp each salt and black pepper

Sprinkle salmon with salt, pepper, and lemon juice. Mix crushed walnuts and parsley, spread mixture evenly over fish and press in.

Toss broccoli and potatoes in olive oil, honey, salt, and pepper. Place salmon, broccoli, and potatoes on a large, foil-lined baking sheet. Bake at 400°F. Transfer salmon to a plate when cooked through (6 to 8 minutes). Continue cooking potatoes and broccoli until tender, about 7 minutes longer.

WHITE BEAN, SPINACH, AND GARLIC PASTA

2 oz of whole-wheat spaghetti
1 tsp minced garlic
1 tsp olive oil
Pinch of red-pepper flakes
¼ cup chicken broth
2 tbsp dry white wine
1 tbsp lemon juice
1 tsp butter
4 cups baby spinach
⅓ cup white beans
2 tbsp grated Parmesan

Cook spaghetti. Drain, saving 2 tbsp of cooking water. In a skillet over medium heat, sauté garlic in olive oil about 1 minute. Stir in red-pepper flakes. Add chicken broth, white wine, lemon juice, and reserved pasta water. Bring to a simmer. Melt in butter. Add baby spinach and white beans. When spinach is just wilted, add pasta; toss to coat. Top with grated Parmesan.

SNACKS & TREATS *(150 calories each)*

If these options don't appeal to you, swap in a 150-calorie snack or treat of your choosing.

PEANUT BUTTER & CHOCOLATE TREAT

Spread 2 tsp of peanut butter on a ½ oz piece of dark chocolate.

ICE CREAM AND BERRIES TREAT

½ cup chocolate or vanilla ice cream (140 calories or less per ½ cup) and ½ cup raspberries.

BROILED GRAPEFRUIT

Drizzle ½ tsp of honey and cinnamon to taste over two grapefruit halves. Broil for 4 to 5 minutes, or until tops are lightly golden. Top with 2 oz of 2% Greek yogurt and ½ tsp of honey.

PARMESAN & PEPPER POPCORN

Toss 3 cups of air-popped popcorn with 1 tsp of olive oil, 1½ tbsp of grated Parmesan cheese, and black pepper to taste.

DANGER IN YOUR RICE

Arsenic in our food is a real public health problem, and Consumer Reports' food safety experts think that it's important to be aware of your exposure to it and choose lower-risk rices and alternative grains.

Consumption of a type of arsenic called inorganic arsenic can raise the risk of some cancers, heart disease, and type 2 diabetes. Rice, in general, has one of the highest levels of inorganic arsenic compared to other foods. Brown rice has more arsenic than white. There is some good news though: Our January 2015 report found rices with lower than average arsenic levels:

White basmati rice from California, India, and Pakistan, and sushi rice from the U.S. had, on average, half the amount of arsenic than most other types.

Brown basmati rice from the areas mentioned above had about a third less than other brown rices.

The FDA recently proposed limiting the amount of arsenic allowed in infant rice cereals. Consumer Reports food safety experts appreciate that the FDA has taken this step, but we remain concerned about the amount of inorganic arsenic in other rice products. We urge the FDA to quickly set standards for those foods as well.

TIP: Rinse rice and cook it in lots of water to lower arsenic content by 30 percent. Try a 6:1 ratio of water to rice.

3 FOODS TO EAT FOR STRENGTH

Want to eat yourself stronger? Research tells us that being smart about your intake of vitamin D and protein is one of the secrets.

Vitamin D. While not conclusive, research has found that vitamin D plays a role in not only preventing muscle loss but possibly increasing muscle strength. The Institute of Medicine recommends 600 IU per day until age 70, and 800 IU after.

Protein. We need daily protein to maintain muscle, and those levels may increase as we age. That's why pumping up your protein intake may be a good idea.

Most experts recommend shooting for 0.4 to 0.7 grams of protein per pound of body weight each day. If you're over 65 aim for at least 0.6 grams. That's 78 daily grams of protein for a 130-pound woman, age 65 or over, and 96 grams for a 160-pound man, age 65 or over.

Your best sources of both protein and vitamin D. Sun exposure is the best source of D but raises skin cancer risk. That's why foods rich in *both* vitamin D and protein are such a good idea. Here are three with that winning combination:

1. Salmon (*preferably wild*)
2. Sardines
3. D-fortified milk

If you're over 65, rarely spend time outside, or eat few foods with vitamin D, a daily 1,000-IU supplement may be reasonable. Talk to your doctor.

THE MINERAL YOU'RE PROBABLY MISSING

Ask most people to name a nutrient lacking in the American diet, and the top answers would probably be calcium, vitamin D, or fiber. But magnesium, an important mineral, is often overlooked.

Though all nutrients are essential for good health, few are more crucial to focus on than magnesium — because we don't usually get enough in our diet and none of our cells could function without it.

HOW MAGNESIUM CAN DRAMATICALLY IMPROVE YOUR LONG-TERM HEALTH

Cells need the mineral to produce ATP, a compound dubbed the body's "energy currency," says Fudi Wang, M.D., Ph.D., professor of nutrition at Zhejiang University in China. That's because ATP is the bank that cells draw on to power their functions.

Magnesium is involved in regulating blood pressure, blood sugar, heart rate, and nerve transmission. But nearly half of all Americans — and 70 to 80 percent of those over age 70 — aren't meeting their daily magnesium needs.

Older people are at risk for magnesium deficiency because they not only tend to consume less of it than younger adults but also may absorb less from what they eat, and their kidneys may excrete more of it. Digestive disorders such as Crohn's disease or celiac disease can also affect magnesium absorption, and people with type 2 diabetes or who take diuretics may lose more through their urine.

MAGNESIUM MAY IMPROVE YOUR LONGEVITY

These shortfalls may contribute to diminished health long-term. In a 2016 review of 40 studies involving a total of more than 1 million people, Wang and his colleagues found that every 100 mg increase in magnesium from food reduced the risk of heart failure by 22 percent, type 2 diabetes by 19 percent, and stroke by 7 percent.

Those who consumed more magnesium were also less likely to die from any cause during the studies' follow-up periods, which ranged from 4 to 30 years.

GET YOUR DAILY DOSE

To get sufficient magnesium, focusing on food is best, unless your doctor instructs otherwise, Wang says. High doses from supplements may have unpleasant side effects, such as diarrhea, nausea, and abdominal cramps, and may prevent some drugs (such as certain antibiotics and bisphosphonates) from doing their jobs. Though no one food has a huge amount of the nutrient, it's not hard to get enough if you keep the best magnesium sources — dark leafy greens, legumes, nuts, and whole grains — in regular rotation, says Joan Salge Blake, Ed.D., R.D.N., clinical associate professor of nutrition at Boston University.

For instance, these foods supply at least 50 mg per serving:

½ cup cooked quinoa

2 tablespoons pumpkin seeds

¼ cup almonds

¾ cup cooked chickpeas

2 heaping cups raw spinach

1 ounce 70- to 85-percent dark chocolate

Magnesium supplements have long been used for leg cramps, but research suggests that pills won't do much to prevent these muscle spasms.

Supplements may be appropriate, however, if you have a

digestive disorder or diabetes. Long-term use of proton pump inhibitors (PPIs) for acid reflux may also lead to a magnesium deficiency.

"MAG" UP YOUR MEALS

Women should be getting 320 mg of magnesium per day; men, 420 mg. Here's a daily menu that supplies just over 420 mg.

BREAKFAST

NUTTY BANANA OATMEAL
⅓ cup rolled oats prepared with water
¼ cup sliced almonds
1 small banana, sliced

LUNCH

VEGGIE TACO BOWL
¾ cup brown rice, cooked
⅓ cup black beans
1 cup sliced zucchini and yellow squash, cooked
¼ cup salsa
½ medium avocado, cubed

SNACK

YOGURT WITH RASPBERRIES
7 ounces low-fat plain Greek yogurt
½ cup raspberries

DINNER

SALMON, SPINACH, AND POTATO
3 ounces wild salmon, broiled
3 cups raw spinach, sautéed with garlic and oil
1 small baked potato

DRUG AND FOOD INTERACTIONS

Some foods — even those that are good for you — can interfere with the way certain medications work.

Eating some otherwise wholesome foods while taking certain brand-name and generic drugs can lead to unpleasant, or even dangerous, side effects.

To get the most accurate information for you, ask your doctor or pharmacist about any possible food interactions with the medicines that you take. Here are four common foods known to cause potential problems.

4 FOODS NOT TO EAT IF YOU ARE TAKING CERTAIN DRUGS

1. *Bananas.* Don't mix with ACE inhibitors taken to lower blood pressure or treat heart failure, and certain diuretics to reduce fluid retention and treat high blood pressure.

What can happen: Irregular heartbeat and palpitations. Taking ACE inhibitors and "potassium sparing" diuretics can lead to higher levels of potassium in the body. When those drugs are combined with large amounts of potassium-rich bananas, the excess potassium can cause heart problems.

Bananas and other foods rich in potassium, such as oranges and green leafy vegetables should be eaten in moderation.

2. *Kale and other greens.* Be cautious when taking warfarin (*Coumadin*® and generic) and blood thinners used to prevent strokes and other problems caused by clots.

What can happen: The drug's effectiveness can be reduced. Kale and other greens (including broccoli and brussels sprouts) are rich in vitamin K, which helps the blood to clot, thus working against warfarin's anti-clotting effects.

There's no need to entirely drop the green veggies from your diet; just don't overdo them.

3. Walnuts and high-fiber foods.

Don't mix with levothyroxine (*Levothroid®*, *Levoxyl®*, *Synthroid®*, and generic) used in the treatment of an underactive thyroid.

What can happen: Foods such as walnuts, soybean flour, and cottonseed meal might make thyroid meds less effective. So can eating a high-fiber diet or taking fiber supplements. If you eat a high-fiber diet, you might need a higher dosage.

4. Grapefruit.

Don't mix with cholesterol-lowering statins such as atorvastatin (*Lipitor®* and generic) and lovastatin (*Mevacor®* and generic).

What can happen: Increased risk of side effects, especially muscle pain. A substance in grapefruit prevents certain statin drugs from being metabolized, leading to higher amounts of the drug in the bloodstream; drinking more than 1 quart of grapefruit juice per day can result in dangerous levels. Whole grapefruit and grapefruit juice can interfere with other drugs too, including certain antihistamines and some prescribed for blood pressure.

PAY ATTENTION TO ALCOHOL WARNINGS

Many medications come with instructions not to drink alcohol while you're taking them. It's an important warning.

What can happen: Alcohol alone can make you drowsy, light-headed, and less coordinated; when it's mixed with certain drugs, those effects can be magnified.

Certain drug-alcohol combos can increase the chance of serious side effects, such as internal bleeding, difficulty breathing, and heart problems. And although alcohol might make a drug less effective, it can also make it toxic. For example, just a few drinks mixed with the pain reliever acetaminophen (*Tylenol* and generic) can damage your liver.

KEEP YOUR BRAIN SHARP WITH THE *MIND* DIET

T he MIND diet may make your brain "younger" and reduce your risk of Alzheimer's disease.

Chances are, you purposely ate something today that you know is heart-healthy, but you probably didn't give much thought to feeding your brain. Only relatively recently have researchers begun to study the link between diet and cognitive function, and the findings are promising.

"You can't control your genes, which are mostly responsible for any decline in brain function as we age, but with diet, there's the potential to do something," says Lon S. Schneider, M.D., a professor of psychiatry, neurology, and gerontology at the University of Southern California.

It takes more than eating familiar "brain" foods such as fish or blueberries once in a while. "It's what we eat as a whole," says Martha Clare Morris, Sc.D., director of nutrition and nutritional epidemiology at the Rush University Medical Center. Research by Morris and her colleagues shows that following a diet that includes the right foods in the right combination can take years off your brain.

The MIND diet is a hybrid of the heart-healthy Mediterranean and the blood-pressure-lowering DASH diets. MIND stands for Mediterranean-DASH Intervention for Neurodegenerative Delay.

The Rush team created the plan after reviewing the evidence from human and animal studies on diet and brain health and singled out foods that appeared to have brain-protecting effects. It limits red meat, butter and stick margarine, pastries and sweets, fried and fast food, and cheese. But a few foods play starring roles. Working these foods into your diet can help keep your mind sharp and your entire body healthy. See 8 Power Foods for Your Brain, page 105.

The Rush team studied the diets of almost 1,000 elderly adults, who were followed for an average of 4½ years.

People whose diets were most strongly in line with the MIND diet had brains that functioned as if they were 7½ years younger than those whose diets least resembled this eating style.

A follow-up study showed that they also cut their risk of developing Alzheimer's disease in half. People who followed the plan only some of the time still had a 35-percent-lower risk. Working these foods into your diet can help keep your mind sharp and your entire body healthy.

8 POWER FOODS FOR YOUR BRAIN

What you should eat to get the benefits of the MIND diet.

1. Vegetables/leafy greens

Eat THIS *At least one cup raw or ½ cup cooked green and ½ cup of other cooked vegetables per day*

It's not yet clear how greens improve brain health, but it may be because of their high levels of vitamin K, folate, and the antioxidants beta carotene and lutein. Research found that people who had one to two servings of greens per day, such as collards, kale, and spinach, for about five years, had the cognitive abilities of someone 11 years younger.

Try THIS: Mix a handful of baby spinach or kale into an almost-ready pasta dish or soup; the heat will wilt it.

2. Nuts

Eat THIS *At least five 1-ounce servings per week*

The brains of older women who ate that amount functioned similarly to those of women 2 years younger according to a study in *The Journal of Nutrition, Health and Aging*. A small study found that older men and women who ate just one Brazil nut daily for six months experienced increases in blood selenium levels and appeared to have better verbal abilities and spatial skills.

Brazil nuts contain selenium, a mineral that helps boost the activity of antioxidants that may protect the brain from damage. One nut supplies all of the selenium you need in a day.

Try THIS: Toss a handful of the nuts (or a chopped Brazil nut) on your salad instead of croutons for a nutrient-packed crunch. Stash 100-calorie snack packs in your bag or desk for the midday munchies.

3. Berries

Eat THIS *At least one cup twice per week*

According to the MIND research, berries are the only fruit that benefit the brain. Women ages 70 and older who ate blueberries at least once per week or strawberries twice per week or more had a brain age as much as 2½ years younger than those who ate the berries less than once per month according to a Harvard study that followed more than 16,000 women for almost 20 years. One animal study suggests that the antioxidants in berries can help activate the brain's "housekeeper" mechanism, which cleans out parts of cells that become damaged.

Try THIS: Frozen berries are just as nutritious as fresh and can cost half as much. Toss frozen berries into a smoothie or heat them in a saucepan and use as a topping for oatmeal.

4. Beans

Eat THIS *At least ½ cup cooked, four times per week*

Eating black beans, kidney beans, lentils, white beans, and others provides a hearty dose of folate, a B vitamin that may play a role in preventing dementia later in life according to a study in the *Journal of the Academy of Nutrition and Dietetics*. Canned beans are fine;

just rinse them before using to remove some of the sodium.

Try THIS: Cook white beans with rosemary and garlic, then drizzle them with olive oil for a rich but healthy side dish. Or snack on hummus or try one of the new bean-based pastas on the market.

5. Fish/Poultry

Eat THIS At least 3 ounces of fish and 6 ounces of poultry per week (not fried)

Both fish and poultry are much lower in saturated fat than red meat. And the omega-3 fats in fish may improve learning and memory by increasing the brain's ability to send and receive messages. Older adults without dementia who ate 3 to 5 ounces of fish weekly for the past year experienced less brain shrinkage, a common occurrence with Alzheimer's disease, compared with people who hardly ever ate fish. "In general, the more fish, the better," says Yian Gu, Ph.D., an assistant professor of neuropsychology at Columbia University. She cautions, however, that people should weigh the possible benefits of fish consumption against the risks of mercury and other toxins that fish may contain. Low-mercury options include haddock, sardines, tilapia, and wild salmon.

Try THIS: Replace tuna with canned salmon (it's often wild) for salads or make salmon burgers. Roll cooked, chopped chicken breast into a whole-wheat wrap with ¼ cup avocado, ½ cup shredded lettuce, and 2 tablespoons of salsa.

6. Olive oil

Eat THIS Recommended intake is daily

The phenolic compounds in extra-virgin olive oil may help prevent toxic protein deposits that can lead to the progression of Alzheimer's disease according to research from the University of Florence. Olive oil may also help reduce inflammation and improve blood-vessel function, two factors that can benefit the brain according to a review of 30 studies published in the journal *Nutrients*.

Try THIS: Cook with it and use it on salads and vegetables.

7. Whole grains

Eat THIS *At least ½ cup cooked grains or a slice of whole grain bread three times per day*

Whole grains, like bulgur and quinoa, were associated with higher levels of brain function in a study that tracked the diet of men and women age 65 and older.

Try THIS: Start the morning with a bowl of oatmeal. For lunch or dinner, toss wheat berries with chopped vegetables, beans, olive oil, and vinegar for an alternative to pasta salad.

8. Wine

Drink THIS *5 ounces a day*

Moderate intake of wine, that's 5 ounces a day, is linked to brain health. But beware of a cup that runneth over. It is worth noting that even the recommended amount should be approached with caution. Adults who averaged more than 12 grams of alcohol per day (about the amount in 4 ounces of wine) had an increased risk of developing dementia according to a study from the University of South Florida. If you're at a high risk for cancer, ask your doctor how much you should drink. See Go Ahead and Wine, page 79.

A Day on the MIND Diet

A day's worth of meals following the MIND pattern looks a lot like a Mediterranean heart-health plan.

There are lots of veggies, nuts, whole grains, and olive oil; some beans, fish, and poultry; and a daily glass of wine. What you won't see much of is red meat, sweets, or fried and fast foods. Remember: Eating this way even some of the time has been linked to brain benefits.

BREAKFAST

1 cup of oatmeal prepared with water, topped with ½ cup blueberries and 2 tbsp chopped walnuts. Coffee with milk, no sugar.

SNACK

1 apple and 1 oz of almonds.

LUNCH

A salad of 3 cups of baby spinach with ¼ cup each of chopped cucumber, tomato, and bell pepper; ¼ cup quinoa, cooked; ⅓ cup chickpeas; 3 oz sliced chicken, cooked; 2 tbsp extra-virgin olive oil; and 1 tbsp vinegar.

DINNER

Grilled tilapia with olive oil and lemon; ½ cup of farro, cooked; 1 cup of string beans sautéed in garlic and olive oil; one glass of wine.

DESSERT

1 cup sliced strawberries drizzled with balsamic vinegar.

CHAPTER SIX

HEAL

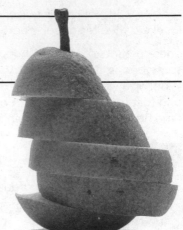

Eat *THIS*
for more disease-fighting nutrients

The healthiest part of pears, apples, eggplants, and even kiwis is in, or just under, the skin. That's where healthful nutrients such as antioxidants and insoluble fiber are concentrated. Leaving the skin intact is usually the best way to preserve the full amount of fiber and vitamins. And remember, it is best to choose organic varieties of these fruits and always scrub them thoroughly under running water.

IN THIS CHAPTER:

FOODS THAT HELP YOU HEAL

For some health concerns, your kitchen may provide good medicine. Here's what to eat and when.

A diet with abundant quantities of produce and whole grains, and moderate amounts of healthy fats and lean protein, can help prevent and control chronic conditions such as type 2 diabetes and heart disease. But certain foods can have a more immediate benefit and may help tame common health problems. So the next time you have one of the four conditions below, consider heading to your kitchen before you open your medicine cabinet.

WHAT YOU SHOULD EAT OR DRINK IF YOU HAVE A HEADACHE, NAUSEA, HEARTBURN, OR INSOMNIA

1. *Sip away headaches with a glass of water.* Whether you have headaches frequently or only occasionally, "the first thing to do if you get one is drink a tall glass of water or two," says Robin Foroutan, M.S., R.D.N., an integrative nutritionist in New York City and a spokesperson for the Academy of Nutrition and Dietetics. "Dehydration is a common cause of headaches, so water may address the pain right away."

Also be aware of the link between headaches, coffee, and other "trigger" foods. Consider, for example, whether you've had caffeine in the past couple of days because caffeine withdrawal can cause headaches. In addition, blood vessels may enlarge during a headache, and caffeine can constrict them, so coffee or tea might offer some relief.

For some people, however, caffeine can set off a headache, so if that happens to you, skip the java. But if you experience migraines, be aware that foods reputed to trigger those headaches — aged cheese, cured meats, chocolate, artificial sweeteners, MSG, and soy — may be to blame much less often than you might think.

"The prevalence of food triggers is really overstated, but people who have them tend to figure it out pretty quickly," says Mark W. Green, M.D., director of the Center for Headache and Pain Medicine and a neurology professor at the Icahn School of Medicine at Mount Sinai in New York City.

"Alcohol is the one exception. It's more likely to cause a headache than other foods, especially if it's heavily fermented, such as red wine," says Dr. Green.

And if you suspect that certain foods bring on your headaches, keeping a food diary can help you pinpoint dietary culprits.

2. *Calm nausea with ginger.* Ginger has been extensively studied as a potential remedy for nausea, especially during chemotherapy and pregnancy.

A 2016 review of research, published in the journal *Integrative Medicine Insights*, found ginger to be effective and safe. It seems to help by moving food out of the stomach quickly and possibly turning off neurotransmitters such as serotonin that can contribute to nausea.

Ginger root, typically sold in candies and capsules, has the most supporting evidence for effectiveness. Occasional use of up to 250 milligrams four times a day is considered safe for most people, including women who might be pregnant.

And don't think you have to stick with rice and dry toast after a bout of nausea. William Chey, M.D., a gastroenterologist and professor of medicine and nutritional sciences at the University of Michigan, Ann Arbor, says evidence does not support long-standing advice to eat only bland foods. He recommends small, frequent meals rich in protein, especially chicken and fish, and vegetable proteins.

"Red meat is hard to digest," Chey says. "There are other proteins that seem to move through the stomach more quickly. Plus they don't cause the same gastric sensations that fats do," he adds. Fats can make the stomach overly sensitive, leading to pain, fullness, and nausea.

3. *Soothe heartburn by eating a banana.*
The typical dietary advice for fighting heartburn and GERD (gastroesophageal reflux disorder) is to eat

Sip THIS

GINGER TEA
Steep 1 ½ teaspoons of freshly grated ginger in 1 ½ cups of boiling water (add honey if you like). Let it sit for 10 minutes, then strain the ginger out before drinking.

smaller, more frequent meals, skip spicy foods, and avoid eating or drinking within 3 to 4 hours of bedtime.

The problem is that it only helps reduce the likelihood of future attacks. Once the burning sensation strikes, try having a banana. Some research suggests that the fruit may act as a natural antacid.

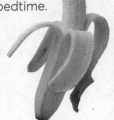

Chew *THIS*

SUGARLESS GUM
Studies have found that sugarless gum may decrease reflux after a meal:

One small study found that people who chewed gum after a high-fat meal had reduced acid levels. Another study showed that people who chewed gum for an hour after breakfast had reduced symptoms for up to three hours.

Also consider cutting back on your consumption of sugar. A small study of obese women, published in the journal *Alimentary Pharmacology & Therapeutics*, found that reducing refined carbohydrates, especially sucrose (table sugar), eliminated symptoms in those who complained of GERD at the start of the trial.

"The diet resolved reflux in all 43 women who had it by week nine or 10, and it wasn't just because of the weight loss," says Heidi Silver, R.D., Ph.D., a research associate professor of medicine at the Vanderbilt University Medical Center and one of the study's authors.

In particular, the study found that every additional teaspoon of sugars increased the odds of having GERD by 13 percent. (Also see Heartburn — Avoid "Trigger" Foods, page 128).

4. Outsmart insomnia with a kiwi snack. Try snacking on two kiwis an hour before bedtime. Recent research published in *Advances in Nutrition* concluded that kiwis may promote sleep because they are a rich source of folate, a B vitamin that may help the brain produce sleep-inducing chemicals.

Kiwis' high antioxidant content may also be a factor. Those plant-based chemicals combat cell and DNA damage from factors such as sun exposure, smoking, and pollution — which have been linked to sleep problems. More research is needed on the kiwi-sleep connection, but it may work for you.

THE MILK-BEFORE-BED MYTH

Some people suggest sipping warm milk for insomnia because it contains tryptophan, an amino acid that is converted to serotonin, which will relax you, and melatonin, which promotes sleep. But studies haven't proved that. Research suggests that sipping milk could help some people because it's a calming ritual.

A TO Z: WHAT YOU *SHOULD* OR *SHOULDN'T* EAT FOR WHAT AILS YOU

 ## ASTHMA

If you suffer from asthma, you shouldn't eat cured meat such as sausage. In a study of 971 adults with the condition, people who ate cured meat four or more times per week were 76 percent more likely to have more severe symptoms over seven years, compared with those who consumed such meat infrequently.

 ## BLADDER LEAKS

There is a link between bladder leaks and constipation because constipation puts pressure on your bladder. That's why if you have bladder leaks, you should be sure to get your fiber. Aim for 3 to 4 ounces of whole grains, 1½ to 2 cups of fruit, and 2 to 3 cups of vegetables per day to keep yourself regular.

 ## CIRCULATION

Try gazpacho. The soup has lycopene and the amino acid citrulline, which some evidence suggests may improve blood circulation. Tomatoes star in this healthy, low-fat chilled soup. Other healing

Try *THIS*

QUICK GAZPACHO

Blend fresh tomatoes and cucumbers, garlic, onions, and fresh herbs in a food processor or blender; for creaminess, add avocado. Stir in cooked corn, fish, or shrimp if you like.

ingredients can include cucumbers, garlic, onions, and fresh herbs. Some recipes even call for watermelon.

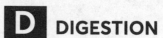 DIGESTION

By now, you've probably heard that a little bacteria in your food isn't always a bad thing. Beneficial live bacteria and yeasts, called probiotics, which are found in some foods, have been associated with many benefits: weight loss and improved digestion and immunity, among others. Benjamin Wolfe, Ph.D., an assistant professor of microbiology at Tufts University, says, "the benefits people get from fermented foods come largely from improved digestibility and the nutrients the foods provide."

Try THESE

3 gut-boosting probiotic foods you should be eating:

1. Sauerkraut
2. Yogurt
3. Tempeh

Sip THIS

Drinking water is a healthy way to help boost energy.

ENERGY

Don't sip coffee or tea in the afternoon. While both coffee and tea can give you a boost, the caffeine can also interrupt sleep later, which can zap your energy. That's why it's a good idea to limit the stimulant to 400 mg per day (roughly two to four 8-ounce cups of coffee) and taper off by late afternoon. Caffeine can disrupt sleep when it's consumed even 6 hours before bedtime.

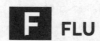 FLU

If you have the flu, you should avoid alcohol. Alcohol is dehydrating, and a flu virus lives longer when the air in your lungs is dry. In addition to avoiding alcohol, drink plenty of water. Also consider using a humidifier to keep humidity at 30 to 50 percent.

GALLSTONES

People can live with gallstones and never know it, but when something triggers an attack, it can be frightening, sudden, and painful.

For example, high fat content of a single meal can precipitate a gallbladder attack in people who have gallstones. Think Thanksgiving feast.

Don't *EAT*

FATTY MEALS
The best way to spare yourself the pain of a gallstone attack is to avoid fatty meals.

You may see advertisements for gallbladder cleanses. They involve eating or drinking a combination of olive oil, herbs and some type of fruit juice over the course of two or more days — during which you may be advised to eat nothing else. However, there is no scientific evidence that suggests a gallbladder cleanse helps or treats gallstones. A better approach to prevent gallstone attacks is to maintain a healthy overall diet with proper amounts of fiber and hydration.

H HAIR LOSS

Deficiencies of biotin, a B-complex vitamin, although uncommon, can cause hair changes including hair loss. If you're experiencing chronic hair problems for no clear reason, talk with your doctor. "If nothing shows up after appropriate testing, because we don't have a good blood test to detect biotin deficiency, it might be worthwhile to try a supplement for three months," says Consumer Reports' chief medical adviser Marvin M. Lipman, M.D.

But remember that dietary supplements are not well regulated and might contain substances not listed on the label or have much less or more of an ingredient than promised.

 IMMUNITY

<table>
<tr><td>

Eat *THIS*

PROTEIN

Getting 30 percent of your daily calories from protein (preferably lean) can help keep your hair in shape.
</td></tr>
</table>

Consume alcohol only in moderation. Though a modest amount of alcohol appears to improve the immune response, too much "turns off genes that help defend us against microbes and turns on genes that make us vulnerable," says Ilhem Messaoudi, Ph.D., associate professor in the department of molecular biology and biochemistry at the University of California, Irvine. In a recent study in the journal *Alcohol*, binge drinkers (women who consume four drinks within 2 hours, or men who consume five) had fewer disease-fighting natural killer cells.

What does moderate mean? One drink per day for women or two for men. See Go Ahead and Wine, page 79, for more details.

 JOINT PAIN

Extra virgin olive oil contains oleocanthal, which has properties similar to nonsteroidal, anti-inflammatory drugs. Researchers say that about 3½ tablespoons of the oil is equal to a 200-mg tablet of ibuprofen.

 KIDNEY STONES

Sip lemonade. Sipping 4 ounces of pure lemon juice per day (or 32 ounces of prepared, sugar-free lemonade) may cut the risk of a return of two common types of kidney stones — calcium oxalate and calcium phosphate. The lemon juice boosts levels of citrate in your urine, which discourages the formation of stones. This "lemonade therapy" may be a possible alternative to traditional citrate treatments, which are often recommended to prevent kidney stones but can cause gastrointestinal symptoms. Don't add sugar, though; doing so can raise the risk of stones.

 ## LDL (Bad cholesterol)

Eat more barley. The fiber-rich substances in barley, known as beta glucans, have been shown to benefit cholesterol levels. Eating barley and barley-based foods reduced levels of LDL "bad" cholesterol by 7-percent over four weeks according to a recent review of 14 studies.

You have to consume about 6.5 grams of beta glucans, the amount in about 3 cups of cooked barley, to get a 7-percent drop in LDL. But smaller servings still help: 3 grams of beta glucans per day could reduce your LDL levels by at least 5 percent.

 ## MUSCLE CRAMPS

Cramps can be caused by deficiencies in calcium or magnesium; if so, increasing your intake of those nutrients may help. And make sure you drink plenty of fluids through the day, especially if you perform strenuous exercise.

 ## NOCTURIA (Urinary frequency at night)

If you find yourself with an aching fullness in your bladder that prompts you to get up during the night to urinate, you may have nocturia. And it's a condition that might become more pronounced as you age. That's because as we get older, the body produces less of the antidiuretic hormone that helps us retain fluid. This results in increased urine production, especially at night. See Don't Drink box at right.

ORAL CANCER PREVENTION

Eat cruciferous vegetables including bok choy, broccoli, Brussels sprouts, and cauliflower. A study in the Annals of Oncology found that just one serving per week over a two-year period lowered the risk of oral cancer by 17 percent. It also lowered esophageal cancer by 28 percent, and kidney cancer by 32 percent. Each type of cruciferous vegetable has different anticancer compounds, so it's best to eat a variety.

P PROSTATE CANCER

Eat tomatoes. A review of studies in the journal *Medicine* found that men who ate 9 to 21 mg of lycopene per day (a medium tomato has almost 4 mg) were less likely to develop prostate cancer.

A red tomato's bright color comes from lycopene, an antioxidant that may help reduce the risk of cancer, heart disease, and stroke.

Don't **DRINK**

THESE 2 BEVERAGES
Avoid alcohol and caffeine before you go to bed, since they are diuretics. Also avoid foods that can be bladder irritants, such as chocolate, spicy foods, acidic foods, and artificial sweeteners.

Try **THIS**

TOMATOES AND MOZZARELLA CHEESE
Fresh mozzarella is lower in calories and fat than some other cheeses, and the fat in mozzarella enhances the absorption of lycopene from the tomatoes. Serve sliced tomatoes topped with mozzarella cheese and fresh basil, or eat the trio on toasted bread.

R ROSACEA

Avoid spicy foods and alcohol — both can trigger rosacea flare-ups — a condition in which certain facial blood vessels enlarge, giving the cheeks and nose a flushed appearance.

S SNORING

Avoid alcohol close to bedtime. And if you need to, try to shed extra pounds. See page 89 for 9 delicious, healthy meals to help you lose weight.

T TRIGLYCERIDES (High)

Eat guacamole. Avocados, the main ingredient in guacamole, are packed with healthy monounsaturated fat, fiber, and vitamins C and K. Researchers found that using avocado instead of other fats appears to reduce elevated levels of triglycerides, as well as LDL (bad) cholesterol.

Try *THESE*

HEALTHY DIPPERS
Instead of tortilla chips, try pairing guacamole with healthier dippers such as vegetables, whole-grain crackers or pita bread, or shrimp. Use guacamole as a side dish or a topping for sandwiches and turkey burgers. You can also add it to eggs, salads, and soups.

U URINARY TRACT INFECTION (UTI)

Drinking cranberry juice is often used as a natural, preventive measure for women who are prone to UTIs. And there is some evidence that drinking cranberry juice may help reduce the chances of getting a UTI.

But, until now, there hasn't been research to show whether cranberries (or cranberry capsules) work as well as antibiotics to prevent UTIs. In a study, women who had frequent UTIs took either cranberry capsules or antibiotics every day for a year.

At the end of the year, women taking the antibiotics had half the number of infections compared to the women taking the cranberry capsules.

However, after a month, most of the women taking the antibiotics showed signs of antibiotic-resistant bacteria in their urine.

That means that the bacteria evolved so that they are no longer killed by certain antibiotics. So, if you did get another infection, the usual antibiotics might not work. The take-away message:

If you have repeated UTIs, antibiotics are more likely to reduce the number of infections you get than cranberry capsules. Since antibiotics do have a downside, you may prefer to try cranberries to see if they work for you.

V VISION

Eat berries. Anthocyanins, a type of phytochemical found in berries, can help protect vision.

W WRINKLES

Drink water. Adequate hydration is recommended to reduce the appearance of wrinkles.

Y YEAST INFECTION

Eat yogurt. The active cultures in yogurt may reduce the likelihood of yeast infections.

Z ZOSTER (Shingles)

Take an oatmeal bath. An oatmeal bath can soothe the itching, burning, and pain caused by shingles.

You can buy colloidal oatmeal bath remedies or make an oatmeal bath yourself.

Probably the most popular method of making an oatmeal bath is to grind the oatmeal into a fine powder and then add the powder into the tub. Using this method may require an extra clean-up step, because the oatmeal can create a thin film in the bathtub once the water has been drained. The "oatmeal bath bag" method below eliminates the clean-up step: The contents infuse into the water rather than being added directly to it.

TRY A D.I.Y. OATMEAL BATH

Place ½ to ¾ cup of oats into a muslin bag, a large coffee filter, or a thin pair of nylon pantyhose.

Make sure the bag is secure. Tie the muslin bag tight. If you're using a coffee filter or panty hose, close it with a rubber band, ribbon or string. The idea is to make the bag secure enough to stay closed and prevent the oats from being released into the bath water and turning it gritty.

Add the bag to the hot bath water as the water runs. When the tub is about half full, toss in the bag. The heat and motion of the running water will unlock the essences of the oatmeal. Let the bath water cool to a comfortable temperature before getting in, and leave the bag in the tub the whole time you're soaking.

THE COLD FACTS

Chicken soup? Honey? Hot tea? We look at the evidence behind 3 popular home cold remedies to find out which are worth trying.

1. *Feed a cold. Yes, chicken soup really works.*
Research from Nebraska pulmonologist Stephen Rennard, M.D., found that chicken-vegetable soup inhibited the movement of white blood cells that trigger cold symptoms. Soup is also hydrating, so it helps your lymph system flush out the virus and loosens mucus so that you can expel it.

2. *Have a bit of honey for a cough.* Three
studies compared honey with one of the following: the over-the-counter cough drugs dextromethorphan and diphenhydramine, no treatment, and a placebo.

Honey proved more effective than no treatment and placebo, and it might be slightly more effective than diphenhydramine at reducing cough frequency and severity.

3. *Sip hot tea for a sore throat.*
When researchers gave 30 cold sufferers drinks that were either hot or tepid, people who sipped hot beverages reported more relief from runny nose, coughing, chills, and sneezing.

Researchers say hot, tasty drinks promote salivation and secretions that lubricate and soothe the throat.

"With a little honey, hot tea can be particularly soothing to a sore throat," says Marvin M. Lipman, M.D., Consumer Reports' chief medical adviser.

HOMEMADE CHICKEN SOUP *IS* BETTER

In our blind taste tests of chicken soup in our test kitchens, we found that none of the canned soups tasted as good as homemade soup. You can cook a tastier one at home with this delicious recipe:

1 chicken breast half, with skin (about ¾ pound)
¼ cup finely chopped shallots
½ cup finely diced celery
1 cup sliced carrots
4 cups low-sodium chicken broth
2½ cups water
½ tsp salt
⅛ tsp marjoram
⅛ tsp thyme
Pinch of black pepper
3 ounces (about 2 cups) cooked wide egg noodles

Place chicken, skin side down, in preheated 4-quart sauce pan. Brown over medium heat for about 5 minutes to render some of the chicken fat. Remove chicken and reduce heat to low. Add shallots and stir briefly (1 to 2 minutes); do not brown. Return chicken to the pan and add remaining ingredients, except noodles. Bring to a boil. Reduce heat and simmer uncovered for 30 minutes or until chicken is tender. Remove chicken and let cool. Discard bones and skin. Dice chicken meat and return to pan. Add cooked noodles. Serve or refrigerate. (Bring refrigerated soup to a boil before serving.)

Makes eight 1-cup servings

NUTRITION AT A GLANCE
Calories 100, Fat 1.5 g, Protein 11 g, Fiber 1 g, Sodium 460 mg

EASE THESE 4 TUMMY TROUBLES

What works and what doesn't for common woes.

Gas. Constipation. Heartburn. Bloating. Eight out of 10 adults occasionally or frequently experience these and other stomach problems. Many turn to over-the-counter medications for relief. While those drugs can sometimes help, they can also cause side effects. Below, 4 tips for treating common digestive complaints.

1. CONSTIPATION — EAT BROCCOLI

About 15 percent of adults say they have two or fewer bowel movements per week according to research published in June 2016 by *JAMA Internal Medicine*.

And the older you are, the more common constipation becomes.

"Contractions in your GI tract slow down as you age, so it takes longer for stool to pass through your colon," says Purna Kashyap, M.D., a gastroenterologist at the Mayo Clinic in Rochester, Minn. You're also more likely to use medication that can exacerbate the problem.

• *Try this first: consume lots of fiber,* which softens and bulks up stool. Women older than 50 should aim for 21 grams daily; men, 30 grams. You can get that from eating a variety of foods. For example, a medium apple (4 grams), a banana (3 grams), two slices of whole-wheat bread (4 grams), ¾ cup of cooked broccoli (7 grams), and a medium potato (5 grams) add up to 23 grams.

If you find it hard to take in that much fiber through diet, supplements that contain psyllium, such as *Metamucil®*, may help. But some research suggests that snacking on high-fiber foods such as prunes might be a better bet.

Note that increasing your fiber intake can initially cause gastrointestinal problems. Start off slow and gradually increase the amount of fiber-rich foods.

- **Also consider: scheduling your bowel movements.** Most people who are regular have a bowel movement at the same time every day. Try visiting the bathroom 30 minutes after meals, when your colon is most active.

- **Be cautious: about taking laxatives.** People with frequent or long-term constipation often turn to OTC laxatives or are prescribed one by a doctor. But in most cases, that's not a good idea. Stimulant laxatives such as bisacodyl (*Correctol*, *Dulcolax®*, and generic) and senna (*ex-lax®*, *Senokot®*, and generic) can cause dependency as well as dizziness, diarrhea, and nausea. And stool softeners like docusate (*Colace®* and generic) may not work better than a placebo according to a June 2016 commentary in *JAMA Internal Medicine*. If self-help steps don't work and you need short-term help, try a laxative that contains polyethylene glycol (*MiraLAX®* and generic) or lactulose (*Cholac* and generic). It's less likely to cause dependence, although it can lead to diarrhea and gas, says Ari Grinspan, M.D., a gastroenterologist and assistant professor at the Icahn School of Medicine at Mount Sinai in New York City.

2. HEARTBURN — AVOID "TRIGGER" FOODS

As you get older and perhaps put on a few pounds, you may find that heartburn crops up more often. The discomfort occurs when stomach acid backs up into the esophagus, the tube that carries food from your mouth to your stomach.

- **Try this first: cut back on foods that seem to trigger the "burn."** That includes alcohol, fried and spicy foods, garlic and onions, citrus fruit, chocolate, and peppermint, says Gail Cresci, Ph.D., a registered dietitian at the Cleveland Clinic. Other lifestyle changes to try are smaller meals, eating at least 2 hours before bedtime, quitting smoking, losing weight, avoiding tight clothes, elevating the head of your bed, and sleeping on your left side.

- **Also consider: OTC antacids for occasional heartburn.** *Rolaids®* or *TUMS®*, or an H2 blocker such as famotidine (*Pepcid AC®* and generic) or ranitidine (*Zantac® 150* and generic) may offer relief. But if you experience heartburn more than twice per week for several weeks, see a doctor. You may have a more severe form of heartburn called GERD, which, over time, can damage the lining of your esophagus and requires stronger medication.

- **Be cautious: about Proton pump inhibitors,** or PPIs, such as omeprazole (*Prilosec* OTC and generic) and esomeprazole (*Nexium® 24HR* and generic).

They can be appropriate for GERD, but only if lifestyle measures or H2 blockers don't help. Long-term use poses the risk of bone fractures, kidney disease, and low magnesium and vitamin B12 levels. They may also make you susceptible to infections, notably C. difficile bacteria that can cause severe diarrhea and in some cases, death. "One role of the acid in your stomach is to kill off bad bacteria," Cresci says. "If you reduce it too much by taking a PPI when you don't need to, these germs can spread."

3. GAS — SIP WATER

Flatulence and belching are equal opportunity offenders, but older adults can be more vulnerable. Because chewing starts the digestion process, dentures that fit poorly, for example, can make it difficult to chew and swallow food, impairing the process, says Stephen Hanauer, M.D., medical director of the Northwestern Medicine Digestive Health Center in Chicago.

- **Try this first: if you're belching,** cut out gum chewing, smoking, drinking carbonated beverages, and gulping down food and liquids. (All of those can cause you to swallow air.) If you have gas or bloating from eating foods like broccoli, cauliflower, or beans, introducing small amounts into your diet over time can help your digestive system adapt. Anytime you increase fiber-rich foods into your diet, like vegetables, beans, and fruit, you should drink more water too, suggests Samantha Heller, M.S, R.D., senior clinical nutritionist at NYU Langone Medical Center in New York City.

- **Also consider: taking an OTC digestive aid** such as *Beano®* when you consume gassy foods such as beans and broccoli. It contains enzymes that help break down hard-to-digest complex carbohydrates.

- **Be cautious: about OTC antigas products** that contain simethicone, such as *Gas-X®*. There's little evidence they help.

4. BLOATING — EAT MORE FIBER

Your digestive tract slows as you age, causing food to stay in it longer and sometimes triggering stomach pain and bloating. That can also be a sign of diverticulosis, a condition in which small pouches or sacs develop in the lining of the lower part of your colon and affect many people over the age of 60. In some cases, diverticulosis can develop into diverticulitis, when the sacs become inflamed and can cause fever, abdominal pain, and constipation, and, if it's particularly severe, a life-threatening bowel obstruction.

- **Try this first: the same high-fiber diet** that helps you stay regular. Doctors used to recommend staying away from seeds and nuts, thinking they might inflame the sacs, but new research shows that's unnecessary. A *JAMA* study of almost 50,000 men found that those foods didn't increase the risk of diverticulitis.

- **Also consider: The low-FODMAP diet.** FODMAP stands for fermentable oligosaccharides, disaccharides, monosaccharides, and polyols — all carbohydrates. Items to avoid on this diet include: dairy, legumes, products containing wheat, honey, and fruits such as apples, cherries, mangoes, and pears. The diet is complicated, so ask for a referral to a GI specialist or a registered dietitian.

- **Be cautious: about assuming that you are gluten-intolerant.** About a third of Americans shun gluten-containing foods according to a 2014 Consumer Reports survey. But you only really need to avoid the protein gluten — found in wheat, barley, rye, and other grains — if you have celiac disease, which affects only about 1 percent of people. Avoiding gluten when you don't need to is a bad idea; you can miss out on high-fiber foods that can help tame stomach problems. You should see a GI doctor instead, who may find that your bloating is due to another condition, such as irritable bowel syndrome.

7 EVERYDAY FOODS WITH FANTASTIC HEALTH BENEFITS

RED BELL PEPPERS *are immunity-boosters.*
Most people associate immunity-boosting vitamin C with citrus fruit. But 1 cup of chopped red bell pepper has more than twice the amount of vitamin C of a medium-sized orange.

Try *THIS:* Slice into rings; sauté each ring in a pan with olive oil and crack an egg into the middle. Cook for about 3 minutes per side.

POTATOES *can lower blood pressure.* Those starchy veggies get a bad rap because of their high carbohydrate content. But purple and white potatoes, rich in the minerals magnesium and potassium, can help lower the risk of hypertension according to a review in the *Annals of Medicine.*

Try *THIS:* Toss cubed potatoes with olive oil, lemon juice, and thyme and roast at 375°F for 45 minutes or until golden brown (toss every 10 minutes).

PARSLEY *has a lot of vitamin K.* A quarter-cup of this chopped herb packs 246 micrograms of bone-building vitamin K, almost three times the amount you need in a day.

Try *THIS:* Sprinkle parsley on eggs, pasta, and soups, or process it with olive oil, garlic, walnuts, and Parmesan cheese for a fresh twist on pesto.

RASPBERRIES *have more fiber than most other fruit.*
A cup of raspberries has 8 grams of digestion-aiding, fill-you-up fiber. A cup of apple slices has only about 3 grams.

Try THIS: Layer with Greek yogurt and high-fiber cereal for a tasty parfait.

PEAS *are a good source of protein.* Green peas are a great source of the nutrient, which builds muscle. One cup has 8 grams of protein, 2 grams more than you'll find in a large egg.

Try THIS: Whirl peas in a food processor with olive oil, garlic, lemon juice, and parsley for a healthful, hummus-like spread.

POPCORN *is a whole grain.* This snack food is one of the most nutritious ones around because it's a fiber-rich, heart-disease-preventing whole grain. Just be careful what you put on it. Loads of butter or movie theater "buttery topping" can pile on empty calories.

Try THIS: Toss air-popped popcorn with olive oil and antioxidant-rich dried spices such as oregano and rosemary.

SAUERKRAUT *is probiotic-packed.* You probably think of yogurt as the go-to source for healthy bacteria to keep your gut in balance. But pickled foods such as sauerkraut and kimchi can also be rich in probiotics.

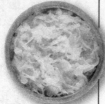

Try THIS: Look for refrigerated sauerkraut that hasn't been pasteurized to gain the full benefits. But young children, people older than 75, and those with compromised immune systems should avoid unpasteurized foods.

MAKE OVER YOUR FRIDGE TO MAKE GOOD CHOICES EASIER

Getting the fridge in shape can mean the difference between selecting foods that heal instead of hurt. A few tips:

• *Rotate the shelves.* Stock up on pepper slices, carrot sticks, cut fruit, hummus, yogurt, and hard-boiled eggs, and keep it all at eye level. You're three times more likely to reach for healthy food if it's on the middle shelf.

• *Store healthy foods in clear containers or bags.* Keep foods you want to eat in plain sight and foods you want to cut down on in the crisper: Out of sight, out of mind.

• *Keep the pitcher full.* Try filling a glass pitcher with unsweetened iced tea or water and adding some cut-up oranges or other fruit, mint, ginger, or cucumbers. Seeing it will remind you to stay hydrated, and adding the flavorings makes plain water more palatable.

• *Spice up the side door.* Stock up on flavorful, healthy ingredients such as salsa, pesto, jarred garlic, roasted red peppers, and artichoke hearts. They're low in calories and fat and can be used as a base for sauces, dips for sliced raw veggies, and toppings for cooked lean meats or fish.

• *Cook, then freeze.* Whole grains and beans can be frozen. Store one or two servings in individual plastic freezer bags. That way, you'll always have a foundation for a quick, healthy meal on hand.

CHAPTER SEVEN

THINK

Eat *THIS*
to help prevent cancer

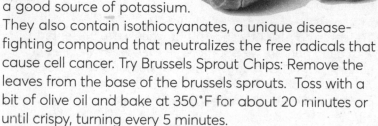

Brussels sprouts are rich in vitamins minerals and are a good source of potassium. They also contain isothiocyanates, a unique disease-fighting compound that neutralizes the free radicals that cause cell cancer. Try Brussels Sprout Chips: Remove the leaves from the base of the brussels sprouts. Toss with a bit of olive oil and bake at 350°F for about 20 minutes or until crispy, turning every 5 minutes.

IN THIS CHAPTER:

THE TRUTH ABOUT PORTION CONTROL

Twenty years ago, a small popcorn at a movie theater had just 270 calories; today, it has 650 calories. And a tub of popcorn these days can top 1,600 calories.

Of course, you don't have to eat the whole bucket. But there's a good chance you'll scarf down at least a large portion of it.

Faced with an abundance of food, we have a hard time saying no according to a 2015 review of 72 studies published by the Cochrane Library.

"Research consistently shows that when we're presented with a big portion, we eat more — even when we are not hungry," says Lisa Young, Ph.D., R.D., author of *The Portion Teller Plan* (Morgan Road Books, 2005) and an adjunct professor of nutrition at New York University.

So can shrinking our waistlines be as simple as bringing serving sizes down a notch? That can help, Young and other experts say. But downsizing portions is only one piece of the puzzle. For weight control — and good health — there are foods you'll actually want to eat more of.

And unless you take steps to ensure that you feel full on smaller portions, your serving sizes will probably creep up again. Follow the techniques below to help you train your brain to recognize and stick with healthy helpings of food.

SMART-SIZE YOUR MEALS
Using portion control as your primary healthy-eating strategy

allows you to eat almost any food while keeping calories in check. And the calorie savings are significant:

> **Normalizing portions could reduce calorie intake by almost one-third — about 527 calories per day according to one study. If all else remains equal, you could lose a pound per week.**

• *Scoop and pour.* Pull out some measuring spoons and cups to dole out precise portions of your favorite foods for a few weeks. You might be surprised to see that a serving of the cereal you eat most days is ¾ cup, while filling up the bowl puts you closer to 2 or 3 cups.

• *Split your dish with a friend.* When dining out, start with your own healthy appetizer, such as salad or soup, and split the entrée. It's also wise to go halfsies on extras, like a side of french fries or dessert. And that might not leave you feeling deprived, especially since researchers tell us that the first few bites taste the best. That's because satisfaction with a food declines with continued consumption of it, a concept known as taste satiety. We're likely to eat more if the portion is large, whether or not the food tastes fabulous. Instead, try having a smaller serving, and slow down so that you can enjoy each bite.

• *Watch your portions of healthy foods too.* Plenty of nutritious foods, such as almonds and dates, are also high in calories. And when people think that a food is good for them, they underestimate calories according to a study from Cornell University. The researchers found that diners who ate in a restaurant they thought of as healthy believed they consumed 151 fewer calories than the meal actually contained.

STAY SATISFIED

Resized portions will seem small only if they're not satisfying. By favoring satiating foods, you can feel full from smaller servings.

Solve the big portion problem

Use your hands to train your brain to make better food choices.

FINGERTIP
Equal to 1 teaspoon; is a portion of fats like mayonnaise or butter

CUPPED HAND
Equal to ½ cup or one ounce; is a portion of cheese or nuts

THUMB
Equal to 1 tablespoon; is a portion of jam or salad dressing

FIST
Equal to 1 cup; is a portion of cereal, yogurt, or raw leafy vegetables

PALM
Equal to 3 ounces; is a portion of cooked meat, fish, or chicken

- **Focus on fiber.** Simply choosing foods that are rich in fiber can help fill you up. Think of how you feel after 1 cup of oatmeal vs. the same size serving of cornflakes. Other fiber-rich choices include beans, fruits, vegetables, and whole grains.

- **Curb your appetite.** Take the edge off your hunger with a healthy appetizer; that will help you limit yourself to that 1-cup serving of cooked pasta. A salad before or during the meal helped people eat 11-percent-fewer calories overall according to a study in the journal *Appetite*. Another study showed that starting a meal with soup can cut calorie intake by up to 20 percent. But stick to a lower-calorie broth-based soup like minestrone or chicken (and check sodium too, because soups often contain lots of it).

- **Take smaller bites.** That can help you keep portions in check. For example, research from the Netherlands found that people who took tinier sips of tomato soup ate about 30 percent less than those who gulped it. (The researchers said that the finding applies to solid food too.)

WHEN YOU *SHOULD* OVERSIZE YOUR PORTIONS

There are a few instances when oversized portions may be helpful — if you're careful.

ONE SIMPLE STEP MAY HELP YOU LOSE POUNDS

EAT MORE FIBER

In a 2015 study, obese men and women who consumed at least 30 grams of fiber a day lost almost as much as people who followed the stricter American Heart Association dietary recommendations. People who simply increased their fiber intake lost 4.6 pounds. People who followed the American Heart Association regime lost 6 pounds.

Sure, the difference is modest, but increasing fiber was the ONLY change they made.

- **Supersize the salad.** It's difficult to find fault with a heaping bowl of raw vegetables. So in addition to the standard lettuce, tomato, and cucumbers, add asparagus, beets, green beans, or whatever vegetables you like. Watch out for the extras, though — cheese, croutons, wonton noodles, and, of course, dressing can catapult a salad's calorie count into double-cheeseburger range.

At a salad bar? Measure out the extras. If you're at a restaurant, get the dressing on the side so that you can control how much you put on. Or just ask for balsamic vinegar plus a little olive oil splashed on top.

- **Eat veggies family style.** Measure out carbs (like potatoes) and protein (like steak) to control portions of higher-calorie foods. But put vegetable side dishes on the table so that people can help themselves to abundant servings of those filling, low-calorie foods. Cornell University researchers found that people eat more of foods that are right in front of them. In the case of fiber-rich, low-calorie produce, you might fill up on fewer calories.

- **Increase portions with produce.** Not sure a half-cup serving of cooked rice will fill you up? Round it out with vegetables. For example, add 1 cup of chopped fresh spinach per serving of rice for a bulked-up but not weighed-down side dish.

Try this: Mix the spinach into the hot rice as it finishes cooking, stir, and cover the pot for 1 minute. After the heat wilts the greens, stir again before serving.) You get a bigger portion — and an extra serving of nutrient-packed veggies.

HIDDEN SUGAR IN YOUR FOOD

You may be eating more of the sweet stuff than you think — and that could be harming your health.

It's no secret that foods such as soda and doughnuts are packed with added sweeteners. But would you think that the frozen stir-fry dinner you had last night would have the same amount of sugars as 16 gummi bears?

Or that whole-wheat bread can have almost a teaspoon of sugars per slice?

These days, food companies toss added sugars into almost three-quarters of all packaged products, including nutritious-sounding items such as instant oatmeal and peanut butter and even foods that aren't supposed to be sweet, like tomato sauce and crackers.

The trouble with sneaky sugars may go beyond excess calories. For example, when 43 obese children ate the same amount of calories but decreased their added sugars intake from 28 percent of their daily calories to 10 percent for 9 days, their weight stayed steady but their cholesterol, triglyceride, blood pressure, and fasting blood sugar and insulin levels dropped.

The study needs to be replicated with a larger test group and with older people, but researchers believe there's no apparent reason that adults would respond differently.

THE DIFFERENCE BETWEEN "NATURALLY OCCURRING" AND "ADDED" SUGARS

Not all sugars are bad for you. Some foods contain "naturally occurring" sugars along with disease-fighting vitamins, minerals and phytochemicals. It's the "added" sugars that can be bothersome. Excess consumption of added sugars has been linked to obesity, heart disease, and type 2 diabetes. Your mission, then, seems simple enough: Enjoy healthy foods with natural sugars and avoid unnecessary added sugars. A few tips to help:

• *Know the code words for sugar.* Ingredients on the list that end in "ose" — fructose, maltose, sucrose — are added sugars (the main exception is the artificial sweetener sucralose). But food labels have a variety of terms for sugars (see 29 Other Names For Sugar, at right). And don't be fooled — healthier-sounding sugars such as brown rice syrup or honey aren't any better for you than other types.

29 OTHER NAMES FOR SUGAR

Dozens of types of sugars can be found on ingredients lists. Here, some of the more common types to look for:

Agave Nectar
Agave Syrup
Barley Malt
Beet Sugar
Brown Rice Syrup
Brown Sugar
Cane Juice Solids
Cane Sugar
Caramel
Coconut Sugar
Corn Sweetener
Corn Syrup
Date Sugar
Dextrose
Evaporated Cane Juice
Fructose
Fruit Juice Concentrate
Glucose
High Fructose Corn Syrup
Honey
Invert Sugar Syrup
Malt Syrup
Maltodextrin
Maltose
Maple Syrup
Molasses
Sorghum Syrup
Sucrose
Treacle

• **Consider the food.** If a product doesn't contain fruit, milk, sweet veggies, or yogurt, and more than 3 grams is listed in the total sugars column, you can assume that most of the sugars are added.

• **Scan the entire ingredients list.** Ingredients are listed in order of weight; the higher up on the list a substance is, the more of it the food contains. But many manufacturers use more than one type of sugar in a product. They are allowed to list them separately, which may give the impression that a food has less sugars than it really does.

THE HONEY BUZZ THAT CAN STING YOU

Just because a product is sweetened with honey doesn't mean it's better for you. The main components of honey are in fact sugars (mostly fructose and glucose), so using too much of it may lead to the same health problems as consuming too much sugar.

Honey is sweeter than table sugar, so less of it is needed to sweeten foods. It contains some proteins that may improve immune function, and it has high levels of several antioxidants.

A bit of honey is fine, and may even offer some advantages," says David Katz, M.D., M.P.H., director of the Yale-Griffin Prevention Research Center. "But keeping total sweetener intake low is the winning formula for health."

- **Compare nutrition labels.** Find the "plain" version of foods such as yogurt or oatmeal and compare the Nutrition Facts label against the same brand's "sweetened" versions. The difference in the amount of sugars between the "plain" version and the "sweetened" version is the added sugars. Here's another sweet tip: Buy plain or regular versions and add fresh fruit for sweetness instead of buying foods that are presweetened.

Eat *THIS*

Natural sugars

Some foods naturally contain sugars, such as fruit, milk, and "sweeter" veggies like sweet potatoes or beets. Naturally occurring sugars found in dairy and fruit come in smaller doses and contain fiber, protein, vitamins, and minerals, which means they don't affect your blood sugar as drastically.

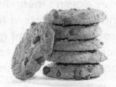

Don't Eat *THIS*

Added sugars

Added sugars are what some experts refer to as "empty calories" because they do not supply any essential nutrients.

SUGAR COMPARISON SHOPPING: HOW TO AVOID SUGAR OVERLOAD

In every aisle of the supermarket, you'll find added sugars in packaged foods and beverages — even in products that sound healthy — sometimes where you least suspect it and in shocking amounts. Here are some ways to sidestep sugar overload.

The American Heart Association recommends no more than than 9 teaspoons per day for men and 6 teaspoons per day of added sugars for women. When you compare similar foods — sometimes even within the same brand — you may find that the sugars and calorie counts vary widely.

COMPARE

BERTOLLI® TOMATO & BASIL SAUCE	VICTORIA MARINARA SAUCE
12 grams of sugars (3 teaspoons) 70 calories per 1/2 cup	4 grams of sugars (1 teaspoon) 70 calories per ½ cup

Yes, tomatoes do have natural sugars, as do veggies such as beets, butternut squash, carrots, corn, and sweet potatoes. That's where the 4 grams of sugars in the *Victoria* sauce come from. But *Bertolli*'s contains added sugars: figure that 8 of the 12 grams of sugar in *Bertolli* are *added*.

COMPARE

CHEERIOS PROTEIN	**CHEERIOS**
17 grams of sugars (4 teaspoons)	1 gram of sugars (¼ teaspoon)
210 calories per 1¼ cup (55 grams)	125 calories per 1¼ cup (35 grams)

Cheerios Protein sounds healthy, but the *Cinnamon Almond* flavor has 13 times the sugars of regular *Cheerios*. There are four sources of sugars in the *Protein* ingredients list. In fact, *Protein* has about as much sugars as *Apple Cinnamon* and more than any other variety of *Cheerios,* including *Chocolate, Frosted,* and *Honey Nut.*

....

COMPARE

MOTT'S® APPLESAUCE APPLE	**MOTT'S® UNSWEETENED APPLESAUCE APPLE**
22 grams of sugars (5½ teaspoons)	11 grams of sugars (3 teaspoons)
90 calories per ½ cup	50 calories per ½ cup

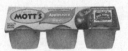 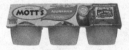

Apples are sweet, but some types of applesauce — like many packaged fruit products — contain added sugars anyway. Always check the ingredients list on canned, dried, and frozen fruits for different types of sugars. *Mott's® Unsweetened Applesauce Apple* has no sugars added, so all of its sweetness comes from the apples. *Mott's® Applesauce Apple* contains about 11 grams of added sugars.

COMPARE

SWEET BABY RAY'S BARBECUE SAUCE

16 grams of sugars (4 teaspoons)
70 calories per 2 tablespoons

STUBB'S ORIGINAL LEGENDARY BAR-B-Q SAUCE

4 grams of sugars (1 teaspoon)
25 calories per 2 tablespoons

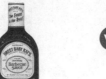

Condiments can contain a surprising amount of added sweeteners. If you choose *Sweet Baby Ray's* sauce, you'll come close to your daily sugar allotment by having just a small 2-tablespoon serving. In addition to barbecue sauce, check ingredients lists on bottles of ketchup, mustard, salad dressings, teriyaki sauces, and the like for added sugars.

COMPARE

AMY'S ASIAN NOODLE STIR-FRY

16 grams of sugars (4 teaspoons)
300 calories per meal

AMY'S THAI STIR-FRY

2 grams of sugars (½ teaspoon)
310 calories per meal)

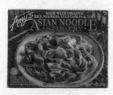

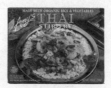

Frozen meals with added sugars? If they have sauces, it pays to check the ingredients list. For example, *Amy's Asian Noodle Stir-Fry* has three types of sugars, including organic evaporated cane syrup and organic cane sugar. Don't be fooled though: "Organic" may make the sugar sound somehow better for you, but it's not healthier than any type of nonorganic sugar.

COMPARE

SCHWEPPES TONIC WATER
32 grams of sugars (8 teaspoons)
130 calories per 8 ounces

SCHWEPPES CLUB SODA
0 grams of sugars
0 calories per 8 ounces

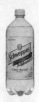

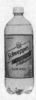

It's called tonic water, but it's really soda — ounce for ounce it has more calories and grams of sugars than regular *Coke*. If you'd rather skip the artificial sweetener in the diet version, try making your gin and tonic with club soda — which, despite the name, has zero calories and no sugar or other sweeteners — and a twist of lime.

COMPARE

ALMOND BREEZE VANILLA
13 grams of sugars
(3 teaspoons)
80 calories per cup

ALMOND BREEZE VANILLA UNSWEETENED
0 grams of sugars
30 calories per cup

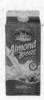

Nut milks and soy milks usually have added sugars, even in the plain versions. But there's a big difference in sugar content between the two here, which shows you that it's a good idea to compare the unsweetened to the sweetened version of a product. If you find the unsweetened version unpalatable, you can add a small amount of sugar on your own.

4 WAYS TO OUTSMART A SWEET TOOTH

1. Reduce added sugar gradually. It's difficult and impractical to erase all sugar from your diet in one clean sweep, so gradually reduce the amount you add to cereal, coffee, tea, and other foods, and gradually start choosing foods with less of the white stuff. Over time, you may find that you've tricked your taste buds into enjoying your morning coffee with just one packet of sugar instead of five.

2. Satisfy your sweet tooth with healthy snacks. The next time you get a craving for something sweet, consider fruit or low-sugar cereal or add your own fruit to plain yogurt.

3. Watch what you drink. While soft drinks account for almost half of the added sugars in the American diet, many ready-to-drink teas and juice drinks are also loaded with sugars. For healthier versions, spike water with a few ounces of strongly-flavored tea, a generous squeeze of lemon or lime, or ice cubes made of fruit juice. Or blend your own smoothies from fresh or frozen fruit, nonfat or lowfat yogurt, and ice.

4. Substitute with spices. Add sweetness and flavor to food with cardamom, cinnamon, coriander, ginger, mace, and nutmeg. Muffins and quick breads can be made with 25-percent-less sugar, and the sugar in applesauce and pie fillings can be cut in half. Finally, try substituting 100-percent fruit juice for honey or other liquid sweeteners.

SHOULD YOU USE A LOW-CALORIE SWEETENER?

A new study suggests that health risks of sugar substitutes may outweigh their benefits — and they may contribute to weight gain.

If you think that consuming drinks and foods sweetened with low-calorie sugar substitutes like aspartame, saccharin, or stevia will help you lose weight, you might want to think again.

According to an analysis published in the *Canadian Medical Association Journal*, low-calorie sugar substitutes may actually contribute more to weight gain than weight loss.

"Ultimately, we found no consistent proof that the sweeteners help reduce weight," says Meghan Azad, Ph.D., a scientist at the Children's Hospital Research Institute of Manitoba and the study's lead author. "And we found at least some evidence that they do the opposite."

While the current analysis was rigorous, its conclusions are still a long way from certain, Azad says. In fact, she says one of her team's biggest findings was just how many gaps remain in the research on low-calorie sweeteners.

For example, the scientists were not able to compare different types of low-calorie sweeteners or say whether the effects of consuming them in food is different than the effects of consuming them in beverages, because no such experiments have yet been conducted.

But it will take time to map those details out. In the meantime, while there's no cause to panic, it's important to think about what you're replacing your sugar with and whether there's a healthier choice to make — especially if you are trying to lose weight.

TOO MUCH SALT? YOUR SALT SHAKER IS THE LEAST OF YOUR WORRIES

Sodium levels are rising, mainly due to supermarket and restaurant food. Here's how to cut back.

The maximum recommended daily intake of sodium is 2,300 mg. Yet, the average person consumes about 3,500 milligrams of sodium per day.

A big part of reducing your sodium intake is realizing where it's lurking. It might surprise you to learn that it's not from your salt shaker. According to a study in the journal *Circulation*, a mere 5 percent of Americans' sodium intake comes from salt added at the table, and only 6 percent comes from salt added during cooking.

THE BIGGEST SOURCES OF SODIUM

By contrast, 71 percent comes from the packaged and restaurant foods we eat. According to a Centers for Disease Control and Prevention (CDC) report, 10 sodium-laden food categories make up 44 percent of Americans' overall sodium intake. (See following page, 10 Foods That Make Your Sodium Intake Soar.)

Sure, having a lighter hand with the amount of salt you put on your food can help. But cutting down on processed, prepackaged foods that already have salt added to them can help dramatically.

FOODS THAT MAKE YOUR SODIUM INTAKE SOAR

These foods are responsible for more than 40 percent of sodium intake

- **Bread**
- **Pizza**
- **Burritos and tacos**
- **Sandwiches**
- **Cold cuts and cured meats**
- **Soups**
- **Savory snacks (such as chips, crackers, pretzels)**
- **Chicken** (See Hidden Salt in Chicken, page 156)
- **Eggs and omelets**

Even just one serving of these foods is high in sodium. Take cold cuts for example. Just two ounces (about two slices) of *Boar's Head Cap-Off Top Round Pastrami* has 600 milligrams of sodium, and one slice of a large Domino's cheese pizza has 620 milligrams. And other foods, such as bread, contribute a lot of sodium to the diet simply because people eat so much of them.

See the next page for some easy ways to consume less sodium.

9 WAYS TO ZERO IN ON SODIUM

Being careful about the food you purchase is the easiest way to reduce the sodium that's hiding in plain sight. Keep these suggestions in mind:

1. Comparison shop. Whatever area of the supermarket you're shopping in, check the labels on several brands of the same item, just like you would if you were comparing sugars or fat content.

Packaged foods can vary widely among brands in their sodium content. Take whole-wheat bread, for instance. One slice of *Pepperidge Farm's* has 105 mg, while one slice of *Arnold's* has 160 mg.

"Once you find a lower-sodium option that you like, stick with it," says Alice H. Lichtenstein, D.Sc., a professor of nutrition science and policy at Tufts University and a spokeswoman for the American Heart Association. "Don't try to do it all at once; just take it one category of food at a time."

2. Take serving size into consideration. "If you will likely eat more than the serving size on the label, you'll want to multiply the sodium," says Maxine Siegel, R.D., head of the Consumer Reports food testing lab. The Percent Daily Value column can be used as a quick check to see if a food is high or low in sodium: 5 percent is low and 20 percent or more is high.

3. Pump up the potassium. Getting enough of this mineral — which is found in fruits, vegetables, whole grains, nuts, beans, some fish, and dairy products — can blunt the effects of sodium on your blood pressure. Potassium and sodium work together to maintain fluid balance in your body, which has an effect on blood pressure and kidney function. When you're eating more potassium, you excrete more sodium through urine. Potassium also helps blood vessel walls relax according to the American Heart Association.

4. Rinse some canned foods. Draining and rinsing canned chickpeas and other beans and vegetables such as green beans, corn, and carrots can remove up to 40 percent of the sodium.

5. Make whole foods a priority. Canned, boxed, and frozen foods can be high in sodium, especially when they come with added sauces and seasoning.

Even healthy foods can be full of sodium when they come in a package. Frozen vegetables with sauce, and boxed rice and grain mixes are often high in sodium. For example, *Green Giant® Original with Olive Oil & Sea Salt Mashed Cauliflower* has 380 milligrams of sodium in ½ cup, while the brand's *Green Giant® Riced Veggies Cauliflower* has just 10 mg per ½ cup.

Cooking with fresh vegetables, whole grains, fresh lean meat, poultry, fish, and dried beans can dramatically reduce the sodium content of your diet.

6. Downsize sandwiches. "With the bread, cold cuts, cheese, and condiments, sandwiches easily can become a sodium bomb," says Siegel. Try replacing mustard and mayo with avocado, roasted red peppers, or even a drizzle of olive oil to add moistness. Choose lower-sodium cold cuts and add just one or two slices. Or make your own chicken, turkey, or roast beef and use that for sandwiches. Consider eliminating the cheese.

7. Taste before you eat. "Even though packaged and processed foods are the biggest sodium villains, reducing the amount of salt you add at the table can put a dent in your daily intake. Many people automatically pick up the salt shaker and season their food before tasting it, when often the food is already salty enough," according to Siegel.

Even a small reduction in sodium can have a big impact on health. For example, if everyone cut their intake by just 400 mg per day — the amount in less than ¼ teaspoon of table salt — it could prevent an estimated 32,000 heart attacks and 20,000 strokes per year according to a study published in the *New England Journal of Medicine*.

8. Speak up when you eat out. Ask your server if there are lower-sodium options on the menu or if the chef can limit the salt in your dish. "If restaurants start getting more requests like that, they may be more mindful about how they prepare their food," Lichtenstein says. The same goes for food manufacturers. Write, tweet, call, or email to let them know you prefer lower-sodium options.

9. Share. Splitting restaurant entrées is an easy way to reduce calories and cut back on sodium at the same time. Asking for sauces and condiments on the side gives you control over how much flavor (and salt) to add.

HIDDEN SALT IN CHICKEN

Salt may be added even before you get the poultry home from the supermarket.

Many cuts of uncooked poultry contain added sodium. To identify those cuts, check the labels.

They must declare anything that has been added to the meat, such as "a solution of water, salt, and sodium phosphate" injected to help keep the food moist, tender, and tasty during cooking.

Meats prepackaged in a processing plant will also carry a separate, nutrition-facts label listing the total amount of sodium per serving. That label is not required on meat packaged at the store.

The amount of injected sodium varies widely: We found chicken breasts with as little as 119 mg of added sodium per 3-ounce serving and turkey breasts with as much as 373 mg, in addition to 40 to 50 mg of naturally occurring sodium.

Those servings supply roughly 7 and 17 percent, respectively, of the recommended daily maximum of 2,300 mg for people who don't need to restrict their sodium intake.

Experts say that people suffering from or who are at high risk of cardiovascular problems, such as high blood pressure, should be reducing sodium in their diet to less than 1,500 milligrams per day.

FAT FACTS

I **f you're confused about fats these days, you're in good company. With research coming in at breakneck speed in recent years, even experts have a hard time agreeing about which fats we should consume, and in what exact proportions, to improve our health and prevent chronic disease.**

Here's what the strongest evidence says about which fats you *should* and *shouldn't* eat.

DON'T EAT *THIS* — TRANS FAT

In the hierarchy of dietary fats, trans fats are the worst for your health. Like saturated fats, trans fats have been found to increase levels of LDL (bad) cholesterol — but trans-fats consumption also has the effect of lowering levels of HDL— the good cholesterol.

And the health risks don't stop there. Trans fats have also been linked to heart attacks, strokes, type 2 diabetes, inflammation, and even problems with memory and cognitive function.

A study compared health data from counties in New York state that banned artificial trans fats in restaurants with counties that did not. There was a 6.2-percent-greater decline in hospitalization for heart attacks and strokes in counties with the restriction.

Previous research has shown that getting just 2 percent of your daily calories from trans fat — that's 4 grams for someone eating a 2,000-calorie-a-day diet — can increase cardiovascular-disease risk by 23 percent.

HOW MUCH BUTTER DOES THAT EQUAL?

Surprising amounts of fat were found in all sorts of foods and beverages. We found that some "healthy" snacks and cereals contain more fat than others, and that some beverages contain as much fat as salad dressing!

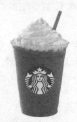
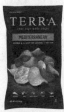
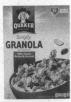

Butter pat = 4 g fat

Starbucks Caramel Frappuccino®
16 oz = 15 g fat

3 ¾

TERRA® Vegetable Chips, Mediterranean
2 oz = 18 g fat

4 ½

Quaker® Simply Granola Oats, Honey, Raisins & Almonds
1 cup = 10 g fat

2 ½

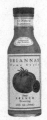

Marie Callender's Roasted Garlic Chicken
1 meal = 21 g fat

5 ¼

Brianna's Home Style Zesty French Dressing
2 tbsp = 15 g fat

3 ¾

Whole milk
1 cup = 8 g fat

2

Progresso New England Clam Chowder
1 cup = 8 g fat

2

With no nutritional upside and plenty of health downsides, experts have determined that there is no safe level of trans-fat consumption.

Even buying products labeled "trans-fat free" or "0 grams of trans fat" doesn't guarantee total avoidance. The FDA allows those claims on products that contain less than 0.5 grams of trans fat per serving. But that can add up quickly if you eat more than one serving or several foods with small amounts of trans fats per day. So for now, the best strategy is to check ingredients lists carefully.

If the ingredients list has "partially hydrogenated oils" that means the food contains trans fats.

LIMIT *THIS* — SATURATED FAT

Found mainly in food such as meat, butter, and full-fat cheese or ice cream, saturated fat can raise LDL (bad) cholesterol

CHOLESTEROL CONFUSION: HDL vs. LDL

The terminology for cholesterol is confusing. HDL stands for high-density lipoprotein and LDL stands for low-density lipoprotein. They are not types of cholesterol, but rather they're fat-protein compounds that transport cholesterol through the blood. HDL tends to carry cholesterol away from the arteries, thus earning the title of "good" cholesterol. LDL tends to deposit cholesterol in the walls of the arteries, that's why it's known as "bad" cholesterol. Sometimes, though, HDL and LDL are used as shorthand terms to refer to the lipoproteins together with their cholesterol cargo.

and increase the risk of heart disease.

And because saturated fat is also found in whole or reduced-fat milk, palm oil, coconut oil, baked goods, and fried foods, we need to watch our intake of those as well.

Heart disease is serious stuff. Nearly 27 million Americans have been diagnosed with it reports the CDC (see box below). What's more, too much saturated fat has been linked to an increased risk of colorectal cancer and other cancers. Recommended daily values of saturated fat when you eat a diet of 2,000 calories a day is less than 20 grams.

HOW TO DRAMATICALLY REDUCE YOUR RISK OF HAVING A FIRST HEART ATTACK

Heart disease is the No. 1 cause of death in the U.S., accounting for 1 in 7 deaths. About 2,200 Americans die of cardiovascular disease each day — an average of 1 death every 40 seconds according to the American Heart Association's 2017 update.

Yet, 90% of first heart attacks could be prevented if everyone adopted a heart-healthy lifestyle.

The finding comes from a landmark study of about 30,000 people in 52 countries. The six changes were:

1. **Eat more fruit and vegetables**
2. **Stop smoking**
3. **Lose excess weight**
4. **Exercise more**
5. **Reduce stress**
6. **Drink a moderate amount of alcohol**

EAT *THIS* — POLYUNSATURATED AND MONOUNSATURATED FATS

Unsaturated fats are the "good" fats. Good fat helps your body absorb vitamins and improve brain function.

And unsaturated fats help protect your heart and reduce the risk of type 2 diabetes. A review of studies by the independent Cochrane Collaboration found that replacing saturated fat with unsaturated fat lowered the risk of heart attacks and strokes.

Good polyunsaturated fats are found in vegetable oils, including soybean oil, corn oil, safflower oil, fatty fish such as salmon, mackerel, herring, trout, some nuts, and seeds such as walnuts and sunflower.

Good monounsaturated fats, are found in nuts; vegetable, canola, sunflower, and olive oils; and avocados. They are also heart healthy, lowering LDL and reducing the risk of heart disease and stroke.

7 oils with high levels of "good" unsaturated fats

| Fat/Oil | Fatty acids % | |
	Mono	Poly
Safflower	14	75
Canola	63	28
Grapeseed	16	70
Corn	28	55
Olive	73	11
Soybean	23	58
Peanut	46	32

Aim for varying your intake of mono and polyunsaturated fats. "We need an array of fatty acids," Maxine Siegel, R.D., head of the Consumer Reports food testing lab, said. "Different acids seem to have different physiological functions." According to a Harvard study that followed people for up to 30 years, replacing 5 percent of daily calories from saturated fat with polyunsaturated fat cut the risk of heart disease by 25 percent. Swapping monounsaturated for saturated fats resulted in a 15 percent drop in risk.

7 WAYS TO LIMIT "BAD" FATS

1. **For breakfast,** top whole-grain bread with peanut butter and sliced bananas or try oat-based, low-fat cereals like Cheerios with a sprinkle of granola for extra crunch instead of bacon and eggs.

2. **Beware of the words "crispy," "creamy," and "tempura,"** synonyms for relatively high fat content.

3. **Avoid salads served in deep-fried shells** or topped with cheese, creamy dressing, croutons, or breaded, fried chicken.

4. **Make your own chips.** Slice parsnips or turnips into thin rounds; toss them with olive oil, salt, and pepper; and bake in a single layer on a cookie sheet.

5. **Make your own sauce** by simmering canned tomatoes with chopped onion, garlic, a little olive oil, and fresh herbs. Freeze the leftover sauce so you can use it in a jiffy.

6. **If you like specialty coffee drinks,** order them with fat-free or low-fat milk.

7. **Keep an eye out for unhealthy oils** in the ingredients: palm oil, palm kernel oil, and partially hydrogenated vegetable oil.

CHAPTER EIGHT

LIVE

Eat *THIS*
to help prevent muscle loss

Many people think they should completely avoid eggs because they are high in cholesterol. But new research shows that the cholesterol in food like eggs has a smaller impact on your overall cholesterol levels than once thought. One egg supplies 6 grams of protein — an important nutrient to help prevent age-related muscle loss and the risk of disability. For example, just one egg helps you reach 10% of your daily protein intake needs if you weigh 160 pounds.

IN THIS CHAPTER:

QUICK SWAPS TO INSTANTLY IMPROVE YOUR EATING HABITS

Think you've heard it all before? These 5 little tweaks will help you turn *good* habits into *great* eating habits.

If you read or listen to the news, it seems that dietary advice is frequently in flux. Should you eat eggs or avoid them, cut back on fat or add another slice of bacon to your breakfast? Look closely at the scientific research, though, and you'll find that for the most part, the pillars of healthy eating don't vary as much as you may think.

One recommendation that has garnered widespread agreement among experts is that a diet that minimizes sugar and emphasizes seafood, legumes, nuts, whole grains, fruit, and vegetables can maximize the protective effects of food.

That's the ultimate goal that many dietitians want people to strive for. But occasionally, nutrition experts make adjustments to that strategy. Here we clarify some long-standing advice that often gets lost in translation and offer suggestions so you can fine-tune your eating to get the most benefit from every bite.

YOU'VE HEARD: Eat whole-grain bread, cereal, and pasta.

NEW THINKING: Eat more unprocessed whole grains.

Switching from products made with refined white flour to those made with whole-grain flours is a good start. But whole grains themselves are better. "They've been tied to so many health benefits, including reducing the risk of cardiovascular disease, stroke, diabetes, and cancer," says Frank Hu, M.D., Ph.D., a professor of nutrition and epidemiology at the Harvard T.H. Chan School of Public Health.

Brown rice, buckwheat, farro, millet, oats, wheat berries, and other grains are considered "whole" because they contain the entire kernel — the endosperm, bran, and germ — so they provide a variety of phytonutrients and fiber and may reduce your risk for certain conditions. (Amaranth and quinoa count as grains too, even though they're actually seeds.) All three components of the kernel are found in some processed whole-grain foods too.

But the data suggest that we should be eating most of our whole-grain servings in their whole form, Hu says. In some cases, whole-grain processed foods contain food additives, sodium, and sweeteners. Ingredients like these may cancel out the benefit you get from the whole grain.

And grains have a lower glycemic index (GI) in their

NOT EVERY MEAL MUST BE BALANCED

You may have read that every meal must be balanced to maintain good health. But your body has enough reserves of various nutrients to thrive for a while if some meals are unbalanced or even missed. For example, foods that provide energy — protein, carbohydrates, and fats —should be replenished daily. Water-soluble vitamins, including the B-complex vitamins and vitamin C, will last two to three days.

whole form than they do in their processed form. That means they're digested more slowly, so they don't cause your blood sugar levels to spike, Hu says. Steel-cut oats, for example, have a lower GI than rolled oats, which have a lower GI than instant oatmeal. Bulgur, or cracked wheat,

VEGGIE BURGERS:
An easy way to get whole grains
These veggie burgers did well in our tests for both taste and nutrition.

PRODUCT

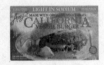

Amy's California Light in Sodium

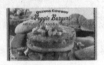

Trader Joe's Quinoa Cowboy With Black Beans & Roasted Corn

Engine 2® Plant Strong® Tuscan Kale White Bean Plant Burgers

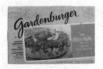

Gardenburger® The Original

has a lower GI than whole-wheat bread.

How to work it in: Grains can go anywhere in a meal. Toss them with beans and vegetables, add them to soups and salads, incorporate them into muffin and cookie batter, or

MAIN INGREDIENTS	NUTRITIONAL INFORMATION
Mushrooms, bulgur wheat	Calories, 110; total fat, 4 grams; saturated fat, 0 grams; sodium, 250 mg; fiber, 3 grams; protein, 5 grams
Quinoa, black beans, red peppers	Calories, 180; total fat, 8 grams; saturated fat, 1 gram; sodium, 280 mg; fiber, 6 grams; protein, 5 grams
White beans, brown rice, rolled oats, kale	Calories, 130; total fat, 1.5 grams; saturated fat, 0 grams; sodium, 15 mg; fiber, 4 grams; protein, 4 grams
Brown rice, mushrooms, oats	Calories, 110; total fat, 3 grams; saturated fat, 1.5 grams; sodium, 490 mg; fiber, 4 grams; protein, 5 grams

serve them plain as a side dish. If you like oatmeal, try a porridge made with amaranth, barley, or millet for a change of pace. Consider whole-grain, air-popped popcorn for a snack. Many grains are high in protein, so they can replace meat if you're trying to cut back.

YOU'VE HEARD: Go low-fat.

NEW THINKING: Opt for healthy fats.

Fat isn't the heart-clogging evil it was once made out to be. But you wouldn't know it from all of the low-fat products still found on grocery store shelves. "Low fat, no fat, and reduced fat became code words for 'healthy,'" says Maxine Siegel, R.D., head of the food testing lab at Consumer Reports.

Yet some reduced-fat crackers, ice creams, and nut butters contain about the same number of calories as the original versions and sometimes more sugar.

And there's an abundance of research showing that certain types of fats are beneficial, even for heart health. "If you get fat from good sources like olive oil, avocados, nuts, seeds, and seafood, that's not going to be a problem," says Hu, who notes that the new *Dietary Guidelines for Americans*, issued in 2015,

TREAT YOUR OLIVE OIL RIGHT

Of all the types of olive oil, extra-virgin should contain the most phenols, that is, natural health-promoting plant chemicals with antioxidant, anti-inflammatory, and anticlotting properties. Heat, air, and light can affect olive oil's flavor and possibly its nutrients, so be sure to buy extra-virgin olive oil in a small, dark colored bottle, and keep it tightly capped and stored in a kitchen cabinet away from the stove and sunny countertops.

no longer suggest limiting total fat intake to 30 percent of total calories. "Those foods contain polyunsaturated and monounsaturated fats, which are the advantageous types in terms of heart disease and diabetes risk."

But it's not all fats; you should still avoid trans fats completely and eat saturated fat — found in baked goods, butter, certain oils (such as palm kernel oil), meat, and whole-milk dairy products — sparingly. (See Fat Facts, page 157)

How to work it in: When you reduce your saturated fat intake, replace it with healthier fats and whole grains for the maximum health benefit. Keep in mind, though, that at 9 calories per gram, fats have more than twice the calories that protein and carbohydrates do, so a little goes a long way.

You can use healthier fats in place of saturated fat for meals that are more filling. Avocado is a tasty replacement for butter or mayonnaise on toast and sandwiches; nuts and seeds add crunch to grain dishes and salads, and they also make satisfying snacks. Olive and walnut oils provide a flavor boost for salads and vegetables.

YOU'VE HEARD: Eat more fish.

NEW THINKING: Eat more of the *right* kind of fish.

Oily fish have an abundant amount of omega-3 fatty acids,

a type of polyunsaturated fat with lots of health benefits. "There's very solid science showing that omega-3s can help reduce inflammatory factors associated with a variety of chronic diseases, including heart disease," says Marian Neuhouser, Ph.D., R.D., of the Fred Hutchinson Cancer Research Center in Seattle.

FISH REALLY IS BRAIN FOOD

A University of Pittsburgh study that tracked 260 older adults for up to 10 years found that among weekly fish eaters, brain areas essential to memory were 4.3 percent larger, and areas associated with thinking were 14 percent bigger, compared with those who rarely ate seafood. Any type of baked or broiled fish helped. For overall health, be sure to choose lower mercury fish.

But, it can be confusing because you've probably heard that some fish are high in mercury. Don't let that stop you from reaping the benefits of fish. The Department of Agriculture's dietary guidelines committee concluded that "for the majority of wild-caught and farmed species, neither the risks of mercury nor organic pollutants (toxic substances that can accumulate through the food chain) outweigh the health benefits of seafood consumption."

The biggest risks come from eating too much of certain kinds of fish: king mackerel, shark, swordfish, tilefish and albacore tuna.

Eating too much risky fish could expose you to potentially high levels of a toxic kind of mercury. In adults, eating high-mercury fish too often might affect the nerves, heart, and immune system. Even low-level exposure in young kids and pregnant women has been linked to problems with hearing, coordination, and learning ability.

A Consumer Reports investigation found that canned tuna is

a common source of mercury and should be avoided by pregnant women. Women who are breast-feeding or may become pregnant — as well as children — should stick to light varieties. White tuna, or albacore, had much higher mercury levels.

How to get the right amount: For a healthy dose of omega-3 fatty acids without too much mercury, aim for 8 ounces a week of farmed or wild-caught low-mercury fish. Stick with clams, oysters, pollock, Alaskan or wild-caught salmon (including canned), sardines, shrimp, and tilapia.

YOU'VE HEARD: Limit cholesterol from food to 300 mg per day.

NEW THINKING: It's more important to cut saturated fat than cholesterol.

Research has found that dietary cholesterol (from food) has a smaller negative impact on serum (blood) cholesterol than experts once thought it did. And setting limits on certain high-cholesterol foods, such as eggs, meant that people were potentially missing out on some important nutrients, says Sandra Procter, Ph.D., R.D., an assistant professor in the department of food, nutrition, dietetics, and health at Kansas State University.

HOW TO REDUCE THE FAT FROM BEEF BUT KEEP THE VITAMINS AND MINERALS

If you pan-fry burgers instead of broiling or grilling them, be sure to pour off the fat. Or try making burger patties in a broiling pan, which has slits or holes to let the excess fat drain away from the meat. If you're going to use cooked meat in a casserole or for pasta sauce, consider first blotting it with paper towels, or rinsing it under hot tap water in a colander and then draining for 5 minutes. An Iowa State University study found that this technique removed half the fat left after cooking but didn't substantially reduce the protein, iron, zinc, or vitamin B12 levels in meat.

"Eggs contain lutein and choline, which are very important nutrients for eye and pregnancy health," she says. A study published in the *American Journal of Clinical Nutrition*, which followed 1,000 men for about 21 years, including some who carried a gene that may make them sensitive to dietary cholesterol, found that eating eggs — up to one per day — didn't raise their risk for coronary artery disease. What does have a greater effect on blood cholesterol is saturated fat, which is why the new dietary guidelines no longer recommend a maximum cholesterol intake but advise keeping the amount of saturated fat you eat to no more than 10 percent of your total daily calories.

How to work it in: Cholesterol is found only in animal products, so when you cut back on them to reduce saturated fat you automatically cut cholesterol. Eggs, lobster, and shrimp are high in cholesterol but low in saturated fat. Experts recommend that you get protein from a variety of sources to maximize your nutrient intake, and those foods can be part of a healthy diet.

YOU'VE HEARD: Eat five to nine servings of fruit and vegetables.

NEW THINKING: Have fruit or veggies at every meal.

Is the salad you had at dinner one or two servings? (Depends on how big it was.) Does the lettuce and tomato on your turkey sandwich count? (Yes.)

Keeping track of servings doesn't have to be a chore. It's much easier to remember that every time you eat — whether it's a meal or a snack — at least one fruit or vegetable should be included.

EAT YOUR VEGGIES FIRST

If you're not eating enough vegetables (and most of us aren't), it could be because you put them in a contest they can't win. "Research has shown that when vegetables are competing with other — possibly more appealing — items on your plate, you eat less of them," explains Traci Mann, Ph.D., professor of social and health psychology at the University of Minnesota and author of *Secrets From the Eating Lab* (HarperCollins, 2015)

"But when you get the vegetables alone, you eat more of them." Mann has studied this strategy — serving veggies solo before the rest of the meal — with college students and preschoolers, but she reasons that it would work for anyone.

"Make a salad and sit down to eat it before you put any other food on the table," she suggests. "You'll not only eat more vegetables, you'll also fill up a bit so that you eat less later in the meal."

"The nutrients, protective effects, and satiety that we get from fruits and vegetables are unparalleled," Procter says. "There are so many benefits, but people just don't get enough of them." Ideally, produce should take up half of your plate. If you're opting for fruit, choose fresh or unsweetened frozen rather than canned fruit in syrup or juice, which has more sugar. For vegetables, there's a renewed emphasis on choosing those that are dark green, orange, or red. Those bright colors are the result of powerful disease-fighting phytochemicals. Legumes, such as kidney beans and lentils, count as both a vegetable and as a source of protein.

How to work it in: Toss veggies into grain or pasta dishes, soups, and omelets. Make smoothies with greens, berries, and avocado or Greek yogurt for a little creaminess. Turn a brownie mix into a healthier option with our Surprise Brownie recipe on page 175. The surprise is spinach, which disappears into the brownie and you get rich brownie flavor with a veggie boost.

BE KIND TO YOUR VEGGIES

Boiling and overcooking certain vegetables robs them of vitamins, minerals, and antioxidants. Instead, try steaming them. Studies show that this cooking method preserves more nutrients in vegetables than boiling, stir-frying, or even blanching them. Use a steamer basket, as shown at right, and a timer. Check spinach and other fast-cooking greens after 5 minutes of steaming; diced or shredded veggie pieces after 10 minutes; and denser vegetables, such as whole carrots or potatoes, after 20 minutes. You can also steam vegetables in the microwave using just 1 to 3 tablespoons of water to preserve nutrients.

Surprise Brownies

½ cup oil

2 eggs

1 (10-oz) package frozen spinach, thawed and squeezed dry

¼ cup plus 3 tbsp water

1 (20-oz) package fudge brownie mix

1. Heat oven to 350° F for glass or metal pans, 325° F for dark or nonstick pans. Grease bottom of a 9x9-inch baking pan with shortening or cooking spray.

2. In bowl of food processor, process oil, eggs, spinach, and water until smooth.

3. Transfer mixture to bowl, add brownie mix, and stir until well combined.

4. Spread batter into prepared pan and bake 34–37 minutes. Add 3–5 minutes for dark or nonstick pans. Brownies are done when toothpick inserted 1 inch from pan edge comes out clean. Do not overbake.

Makes about 20 brownies

NUTRITION AT A GLANCE
Calories 170, Fat 8 g, Protein 2 g,
Sodium 115 mg

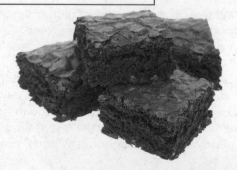

WHY YOU SHOULD THINK TWICE ABOUT A GLUTEN-FREE DIET

It's one of the biggest trends in the food world, but will going gluten free really make you healthier? Here's the reality behind the claims.

"Gluten free" is a claim you see on everything from potato chips to bread to hummus — and even on cosmetics and laundry detergent.

Just as fat was vilified in the 1990s and carbs have been scorned more recently, gluten — a protein found in wheat, barley, and rye — has become a dietary villain, blamed for everything from forgetfulness to joint pain and weight gain.

One piece of good news: A new study in the *British Medical Journal (BMJ)* reveals that for most people, eating gluten is not, as some believe, linked to a higher risk of heart disease.

In fact, unless you have celiac disease, going gluten-free might actually harm your heart, reports Andrew Chan, M.D., M.P.H., associate professor of medicine at Harvard Medical School and one of the study's authors.

"When you start to restrict gluten, you may start to restrict foods that are high in whole grains," Chan says. "Whole grains are linked to better cardiovascular health outcomes."

Celiac disease is an autoimmune condition affecting about 1 percent of people in the U.S. With celiac disease, gluten causes inflammation and damage in the intestine. Some research suggests that the disease may also increase inflammation throughout the body, possibly raising heart disease risk in people with celiac disease. But this *BMJ* study provides evidence that this is not the case for people who don't have the condition.

The research team, from Harvard University and Columbia University, reviewed data on 64,714 women and 45,303 men without celiac disease who reported on their food habits every four years from 1986 through 2010.

In the study, the researchers found that people without celiac disease whose diets contained the most gluten were no more likely to have developed heart disease than those who ate the least gluten.

They also found that avoiding food with gluten was linked to eating fewer whole grains.

The results aren't surprising according to Alice H. Lichtenstein, D.Sc., a professor of nutrition science and policy at Tufts University who wasn't involved with the study. She says there's no good theoretical reason why eating foods with gluten would be related to heart disease in people without celiac.

WHO SHOULD GO GLUTEN-FREE?

A gluten-free diet is a must for people diagnosed with celiac disease. But in recent years, the number of people without celiac disease following a gluten-free diet has grown considerably, with surveys suggesting that about 30 percent of Americans are trying to minimize or avoid gluten. (See box, Do You Have Celiac Disease? page 178.)

Some people who don't have celiac disease do report gastrointestinal symptoms caused by gluten — a condition known as non-celiac gluten sensitivity, which scientists don't fully understand.

Many people self-diagnose themselves with celiac disease. If that diagnosis is wrong, it can lead to starting a gluten-free diet inappropriately.

If you're convinced that you have a problem with gluten, see a specialist to get a blood test to check for certain antibodies associated with celiac disease. You need to be eating gluten when the test is done to get a proper diagnosis, notes Peter Green, M.D., director of the Celiac Disease Center at Columbia University Medical Center in New York. If it's positive, then you should have an endoscopic biopsy of your small intestine to check for damage.

But there's little evidence for the claims that gluten can cause obesity, joint pain, low energy, depression, and migraines in people.

Chan says the results of the *BMJ* study should make people without celiac disease think twice before going gluten-free.

"We want people to be cautious about taking on extreme diets without knowing what the full implications of those diets may be," he says.

THE DOWNSIDE OF A GLUTEN-FREE DIET

It is concerning that people on a gluten-free diet may be eating fewer whole grains, says Lichtenstein — mainly because of whole grains' high fiber content.

Also, she points out, gluten free foods can have more salt, sugar, and fat, and they're often more expensive than their gluten-containing counterparts. "From a straight nutrition perspective, there doesn't seem to be an advantage to choosing gluten-free products," she says. Consider these four points:

1. *Going gluten-free isn't more nutritious — and may be less so.* In a survey by the Consumer Reports National

Research Center, a quarter of Americans thought gluten-free foods have more vitamins and minerals than other foods.

But a Consumer Reports review of 81 products free of gluten across 12 categories revealed that they're a mixed bag in terms of nutrition.

"If you go completely gluten-free without the guidance of a nutritionist, you can develop deficiencies pretty quickly," warns Laura Moore, R.D., a dietitian at the University of Texas School of Public Health in Houston. Many gluten-free foods aren't enriched or fortified with nutrients such as folic acid and iron; the products that contain wheat flours are.

And it may come as a surprise to learn that ditching gluten often means adding sugar and fat. "Gluten adds oomph to foods — wheat, rye, and barley all have strong textures and flavors," says Angela Lemond, a registered dietitian nutritionist in Dallas and a spokeswoman for the Academy of Nutrition and Dietetics. Take it out of food that usually contains it, and you might find that extra fat, sugar, or sodium have been used to compensate for the lack of taste.

2. You might gain weight if you go gluten-free. While our survey showed that more than a third of Americans think that going gluten free will help them slim down, there's no evidence that doing so is a good weight-loss strategy. In fact, the opposite is often true.

In a review of studies on nutrition and celiac disease published in the *Journal of Medicinal Food*, researchers said that a gluten free diet "seems to increase the risk of overweight or obesity." The authors attributed that to the tendency for gluten-free foods to have more calories, sugars, and fat than their regular counterparts. People who have celiac disease often gain weight when they go gluten free, notes Alessio Fasano, M.D., director of the Center for Celiac Research at

If you must cut out gluten, be sure to do it the healthy way:

Eat a variety of grains.
Whether you're on a gluten-free diet or not, eating a variety of grains is healthy, so don't cut out whole grains. Replace wheat with amaranth, corn, millet, quinoa, teff, and the occasional serving of rice.

Shop the grocery store perimeter. Stick with naturally gluten-free whole foods: fruit, vegetables, lean meat and poultry, fish, most dairy, legumes, some grains, and nuts.

Read the label! Minimize your intake of packaged foods made with refined rice or potato flours; choose those with no-gluten, non-rice whole grains instead. Whenever you buy processed foods, keep an eye on the sugar, fat, and sodium content of the product.

Massachusetts General Hospital in Boston. That's because the damage gluten does to their small intestine prevents them from digesting food properly. Their digestive system heals after they have given up gluten and they're able to absorb key vitamins and nutrients from the foods they eat, including calories.

What about those who say they got rid of their belly when they ditched the wheat? There's no evidence that it was due to cutting gluten. "If people lose weight on a gluten-free diet, it might be because they're cutting calories, eating less processed food or sweets, or cutting portions of starchy foods like pasta and bread," says Samantha Heller, M.S., R.D., a senior clinical nutritionist at NYU Langone Medical Center. "Instead of a cookie, they're eating an apple. Instead of pasta, they're eating a high-fiber, gluten-free whole grain like quinoa. Eating more fiber helps satiety and may aid in weight loss."

3. You might miss a serious health condition. "We commonly see patients who go on a gluten-free diet and feel better for a week or two," explains Joseph Murray, M.D., a gastroenterologist at the Mayo Clinic. "It may be the placebo effect or simply because they're eating less. For some, their symptoms come back, so they decide to drop another food group, and then a few weeks later, when they're still not feeling any better, they make an even more drastic change, like going completely vegan. By the time they enter my office, they're on a severely restricted diet and still have symptoms."

The reason? It often turns out their condition wasn't celiac disease or even gluten sensitivity at all, but another condition such as irritable bowel syndrome.

4. You may increase your intake of arsenic and other heavy metals by going gluten-free. Cereals, crackers, pastas and other gluten-free products are often made with rice flour.

Consumer Reports' food safety experts have found that rice and rice-based products can have concerning amounts of arsenic and recommend minimizing your intake of them. A recent study published in the journal Epidemiology showed that people on a gluten-free diet had twice the amount of arsenic and 70-percent-more mercury in their urine than people who were not. (See Danger in Your Rice, page 95.)

"This study provides strong evidence that consumers on a gluten-free diet are exposed to a much higher level of arsenic, as a result of eating products that typically contain rice flour," says James Rogers, Ph.D., Director of Food Safety and Research at Consumer Reports. "This new data, in addition to Consumer Reports' own investigations into rice and arsenic, indicates that consumers should consider trading rice for alternative grains at least some of the time."

GET YOUR GRAINS

Everyone needs to eat whole grains: 3 to 4 ounces per day for most adults. And if you're following a gluten-free diet, pay special attention to including whole grains in your diet, Lichtenstein says. Double check the nutrition label, she says. "Whatever the product is that you choose," she says, "make sure that it's made with the whole grain and not the refined grain."

Ideally, she says, the whole grain will be the first on the ingredients list, since those lists are organized from greatest amount to least amount by weight in the food.

Many whole grains don't contain any gluten. They include amaranth, brown rice (in limited amounts because of arsenic concerns), buckwheat, oats, quinoa, sorghum, and teff. If you have celiac disease, be sure to look for gluten-free labels on products because the grains may be processed on the same equipment as wheat or other gluten-containing grain products.

GLUTEN MAY ACTUALLY BE GOOD FOR YOU

There's some evidence that the protein has beneficial effects on triglycerides and may help blood pressure.

The fructan starches in wheat also support healthy bacteria in your digestive system, which in turn may reduce inflammation and promote health in other ways. One small study found that healthy people who followed a gluten free diet for a month had significantly lower levels of healthy bacteria.

MOVE OVER, KALE

The leafy green's relatives are making a comeback in nutritional circles. Here are a few delicious ways to benefit.

Kale has had a long run in the health-food limelight. Now its cousins — including bok choy, broccoli, brussels sprouts, and especially cauliflower — are being touted as the coolest vegetables on the block.

But to scientists and nutritionists, this family of vegetables, called crucifers, has always been hot. "Cruciferous vegetables are among the most nutritious because they are rich in several vitamins and minerals, plus they contain unique disease-fighting compounds," says Maxine Siegel, R.D., who heads Consumer Reports' food-testing lab.

BENEFITS FOR YOUR BODY

Cruciferous vegetables are the most common dietary sources of glucosinolates. These are natural chemicals that give the veggies their pungent flavor and break down into cancer-protecting compounds. A study in the Annals of Oncology found that just one serving per week over a two-year period lowered the risk of breast, colon, and oral cancer by 17 percent; esophageal cancer by 28 percent; and kidney cancer by 32 percent. Each type of vegetable has different anticancer compounds, so it's best to eat a variety. This vegetable family stands out for its rich bounty of vision-protecting carotenoids as well as fiber, folate, potassium, and vitamins C, E, and K.

Some of these nutrients may contribute to that cancer-fighting ability, and they may also be part of the reason crucifers help control inflammation and protect against heart disease. In an analysis of 134,796 people, researchers in China found that those who ate about 6 ounces per day reduced their risk of heart disease by about 20 percent compared with those who ate an ounce or less.

COOKING AND SERVING TIPS

• *Steam or stir-fry.* These methods preserve the most glucosinolates. Aim for an al dente texture. Overcooking not only turns these vegetables an unappetizing color but also makes them mushy, gives them a stronger flavor than you might like, and diminishes the nutrient content.

• *Make a slaw.* Season thinly sliced raw cabbage with rice-wine vinegar and olive oil. Use as a topping for fish tacos. Test-tube studies suggest that cabbage's sulfur compounds make the selenium in fish a more potent cancer fighter.

• *Hang on to broccoli leaves and stems.* Peel stalks and slice into coins to use in pasta dishes or as a dipper for hummus. Sauté greens with garlic in olive oil.

• *Use watercress for more than a garnish.* Mix it with milder greens like baby spinach and pair with sweet and creamy flavors like avocado and apple slices to balance out the strong flavor.

• *Add cruciferous vegetables to lots of recipes.* For example, give your macaroni and cheese recipe a nutritious and delicious makeover by adding cauliflower. See our Mac-and-Cheese with Cauliflower recipe on page 185.

Mac-and-Cheese with Cauliflower

1 pound elbow-shaped pasta
½ head cauliflower, trimmed and cut into small florets
2 slices whole-wheat bread
1 tbsp olive oil
4 tbsp grated Parmesan cheese
8 oz sharp cheddar cheese, grated
4 oz low-fat cream cheese
½ cup fat-free half and half
½ tsp salt
½ tsp freshly ground black pepper

1. Heat oven to 350° F.

2. Bring large pot of water to boil. Add pasta and cauliflower and cook according to the pasta-package instructions.

3. Meanwhile, pulse bread, olive oil, and 1 tablespoon of the Parmesan cheese in a food processor until coarse crumbs form. Set aside.

4. After pasta and cauliflower are cooked, reserve ½ cup of the cooking water. Drain pasta and cauliflower. Place cheddar cheese, cream cheese, 3 tablespoons Parmesan cheese, half and half, salt, and pepper in the pasta cooking pot. Add pasta and cauliflower. Stir until well combined and cheese is melted. Add reserved cooking liquid.

5. Place in greased 9x13-inch baking dish. Top with bread crumb mixture. Bake until bubbling and the crumbs are browned, about 15 to 20 minutes. *Serves 8*

> **NUTRITION AT A GLANCE**
> Calories 410, Fat 15 g, Protein 17 g, Fiber 3 g,
> Sodium 480 mg

HOW TO TELL IF YOUR FOOD IS STILL FRESH

Have you noticed that some of the jars, cans, and tubes in your pantry have been there for — eons? Use this guide to know if you should or shouldn't eat it.

Foods are labeled to indicate when they should be tossed, although dates can be confusing.

For example, in most cases, eating food that has been on the shelf — or even in the fridge — past the date on the package won't put you at high risk for food-borne illnesses, says Ben Chapman, Ph.D., a food safety specialist and assistant professor at North Carolina State University in Raleigh.

Then why are best-by, sell-by, use-by, and other dates plastered all over food packaging? "Most consumers don't realize that they're really more about food quality than food safety," says Robert Gravani, Ph.D., professor of food science at Cornell University and co-creator of the Department of Agriculture's USDA FoodKeeper app.

A food may not be at its peak after the date on the package, but staleness, color changes, and the like are quality problems, not safety concerns. Foods may develop mold, become rancid, or spoil in other ways, but they are likely to look, smell, and taste disgusting before they become unsafe. When it comes to safety, though, you can't automatically assume that chicken or ground beef is guaranteed not to contain harmful bacteria before the label date. The truth is, the bugs responsible for the annual 48 million illnesses and

3,000 deaths from food-borne pathogens don't cause spoilage. If they're in a food, they'll be there even when it's fresh. And unlike mold, sliminess, and other signs of spoilage, you can't see or smell them.

DEFINING DATES

The federal government doesn't require foods except for infant formula to carry a date label, and the concern for baby food is nutrients, not safety. Several states have regulations, but the guidelines used to set the dates and the meaning of terms vary from state to state. To help consumers, the USDA offers these general definitions:

• ***"Sell by."*** Manufacturers suggest that retailers remove the product from shelves by this date. The goal: to assure quality for a period of time after the consumer buys it. That can be several days to several weeks, depending on the food. For instance, milk, assuming proper refrigeration, should last five to seven days past the sell-by date before turning sour.

• ***"Best by" and "use by."*** These terms tell the consumer when to eat (or freeze) a food for best quality. For example, a jar of salsa may not taste as fresh and tangy as it's supposed to, or crackers may be soft instead of crisp after these dates. But in the majority of cases, manufacturers decide on the terms and dates — based on their own product testing. According to a report from the Natural Resources Defense Council and Harvard University, manufacturers use a number of methods, such as lab tests and taste testing, to set them, but consumers have no way of knowing how the dates were determined. In many cases, the dates are conservative, and you may notice no quality difference — especially if the date recently passed. They're better used as general suggestions, not hard-and-fast deadlines according to Gravani, so if something you have at home is past the date, don't be so quick to toss it.

5 FOOD TIPS TO HELP YOU STAY SAFE

1. *Watch out for mold.* Some types cause allergies or respiratory problems; others can produce mycotoxins that can make you sick. Even if the mold is in one spot, discard the food. Skip the sniff test; certain spores can be inhaled. There are some exceptions. Surface mold on hard salami and dry-cured country hams can be scrubbed off. Also, for hard cheeses (such as cheddar and Parmesan), firm vegetables (such as bell peppers and carrots), and cheeses made with mold (such as Gorgonzola), you can cut off the mold and about an inch around it and use the rest of the food.

2. *Know how to battle the bad bugs.* Keep raw meat cold (37°F or colder) and cooked meat warm (140°F or warmer) to prevent bacterial growth. Defrost meat in the fridge, cook thoroughly, and refrigerate leftovers within 2 hours. Don't let raw meat or its juices touch other foods, and wash your hands, cutting boards, and utensils in warm, soapy water.

3. *Use a meat thermometer.* Tricks such as wiggling the turkey leg, checking the color of roast beef, and piercing chicken with a fork to see whether the juices run clear are unreliable. You need to be sure that meat has reached a safe temperature: 145°F for beef roasts, pork roasts, and fresh ham (140°F for precooked hams that you reheat), and 165°F for chicken and turkey.

4. *Consider avoiding certain foods.* "Refrigeration slows the growth of most pathogens, such as E. coli, norovirus, or salmonella, but not listeria," Chapman says. Deli meat is a top source of listeria. The meat may not contain enough of the bacteria to make you sick when you first buy it, but the bacteria multiply with time, so you want to eat it within a few days. Older adults, pregnant women, and people with weakened immune systems are more susceptible to listeria infection, and the USDA recommends that they avoid eating deli meats and hot dogs unless those foods first reach a temperature of 165°F. Ready-to-eat refrigerated foods, smoked seafood, pâtés, meat spreads, and blue-veined and soft cheeses such as Brie, feta, and queso fresco are also risky.

5. Use your eyes and nose. Regardless of the package date, avoid food that's obviously spoiled. (See the chart on the next page.) If your eyesight or sense of smell can't be trusted, have a friend or family member check out the food for you, or simply discard it when you're in doubt. Never taste a food that you suspect has gone bad.

Time to toss it?

Use these storage guidelines based on advic

FOOD	STORAGE TIME FOR BEST QUALITY	WHEN TO TOSS IT
EGGS*	3–5 weeks	Odd color or odor when cracked
MILK*	1 week	Odd odor or separation
YOGURT*	1–2 weeks	Mold or odd odor
HARD CHEESE* (cheddar. Parmesan)	6 months unopened, 3–4 months after opening	Significant mold. odd odor, sliminess
SOFT CHEESE such as Brie and chèvre (goat cheese)*	1–2 weeks	Mold (excluding natural mold that's part of the cheesemaking process), odd odor, sliminess
CREAM CHEESE*	2 weeks	Mold or odd odor
POULTRY*	Raw: 1–2 days Cooked: 3–4 days	Odd color or odor, slimy or sticky flesh
MEAT (beef, lamb, pork, veal)*	Raw: 3–5 days Cooked: 3–4 days	Odd color or odor, slimy or sticky flesh
GROUND MEAT or POULTRY*	Raw: 1–2 days Cooked: 3–4 days	Odd color or odor, sliminess
SEAFOOD*	Raw: 1–2 days Cooked: 3–4 days	Odd color or odor (a strong fishy odor is bad)
DELI MEATS*	3–5 days	Odd color or odor, sliminess

rom the USDA.

FOOD	STORAGE TIME FOR BEST QUALITY	WHEN TO TOSS IT
HIGH-ACID CANNED FOODS such as tomatoes and sauerkraut	12–18 months on the shelf; 5–7 days in the fridge after opening	Bulging, dented, corroded or punctured can; broken seal; bubbles rising to the surface; liquid spurting out or odd odor upon opening
LOW-ACID CANNED GOODS such as meat, vegetables, and most soups	2–5 years on the shelf; 3–4 days in the fridge after opening	Bulging, dented, corroded or punctured can; broken seal; bubbles rising to the surface; odd color or odor; liquid spurting out or odd odor or color upon opening
RICE OR DRIED PASTA	2 years on the shelf, 3–4 days in the fridge after cooking	Mold, bugs
FRUITS AND VEGETABLES	Varies from 3 days to a few weeks	Mold, discoloration, or odd odor
COOKING OIL	3–5 months after opening	Rancid odor
SALAD DRESSING	10–12 months on the shelf, 1–3 months if refrigerated after opening	Mold or odor

*Store in the refrigerator

CHAPTER NINE

ENJOY

Eat *THIS*

to satisfy a craving

Craving fast food? A fast-food fix doesn't have to be a dietary disaster. *Taco Bell's Fresco Soft Tacos* are on the small side, but you can eat two and still be far better off nutritionally than if you picked — surprisingly — the *Fiesta Taco Salad*. Two *Fresco Soft Tacos (chicken)* have just 300 calories and 12 grams of fat compared to a *Fiesta Taco Salad (chicken)* with 720 calories and 33 grams of fat.

IN THIS CHAPTER:

HOW TO EAT HEALTHY AND HAPPY ALL YEAR LONG

Winter, spring, summer, fall, each brings it's own unique blend of tasty foods — along with some nutritional pitfalls. Here's a breakdown of simple, easy-to-follow health and nutrition advice to help you make the most of each season.

WINTER
How to eat healthy at a Super Bowl Party

Ah, the Super Bowl! Perhaps the first post-holiday event that may sabotage a New Year's resolution to eat better.

"While it's a special occasion, it's important to still be mindful of what and how much you're eating," says Maxine Siegel, R.D., who heads Consumer Reports' food-testing lab. "We just came off the holidays and the overindulgence that went with them... so you should choose wisely."

That can be difficult, though, when you're faced with a tempting array of snacks such as hot wings, chilled brews, and crunchy chips. If the foods you eat at the party will serve as dinner, aim for roughly 500 to 700 calories if you follow a 2,000 calorie-per-day diet. To help you out, we've calculated what 100 calories of common Super Bowl foods look like as a visual guide to help you keep your snacking in check. (See page 195.) And try these 6 tips:

1. *Eat before the game.* Skipping breakfast and lunch to save calories isn't a great idea. You'll arrive at the party starving, and it's easy to go overboard on Super Bowl food when you're hungry.

2. Survey the spread before you make a move. At the party, look over the food choices before you fill your plate. Take a healthy helping from the crudité platter and choose smaller portions of wings, pizza, or other high-calorie foods.

3. Be careful with dips. Guacamole and hummus are loaded with healthful nutrients and are rich in good fats, but the calories add up fast. Salsa, on the other hand, has one-fifth the calories.

4. Skip the chips. You can have a heck of a lot more popcorn and carrots for the same calories you'd get in five corn chips.

5. Don't order the stuffed or deep-dish pizza. If you're ordering pizza, remember that stuffing a large *Pizza Hut* crust with cheese adds about 20 calories, 2 grams of fat, and 100 milligrams of sodium per slice. And speaking of cheese, we don't have to tell you that the words "extra," "double," and "triple" boost calories, fat, and sodium.

A NOT-SO-SKINNY SURPRISE

It's called *SkinnyPop*. Given its name, you might well think that *SkinnyPop* is lower in calories and fat than other brands. But we compared *SkinnyPop* to four other brands of popcorn: *Angie's BOOMCHICKAPOP Sea Salt; Smartfood Delight® Sea Salt; Cape Cod Seaside Pop Sea Salt and Popcorn, Indiana Sea Salt* — and we learned this: *SkinnyPop* had slightly more calories and fat than all of those brands. On its website the company defines "skinny" not as diet-friendly but as "using the fewest, cleanest, and simplest ingredients possible."

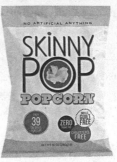

Also, opting for the thin-crust version, when available, usually saves you calories. At *Papa John's*, you'll cut 80 calories per large slice of a cheese pizza. At *Domino's®*, a large thin-crust slice has about 60 fewer calories than a regular hand-tossed slice.

6. Try one of our Super Bowl recipes for a crowd.

No matter which team you're rooting for on Super Bowl Sunday, you'll want your party guests to be cheering for the food you've cooked up. But crowd-pleasing party food isn't always healthy. Help is here with some better-for-you Super Bowl Recipes for a crowd. See page 196.

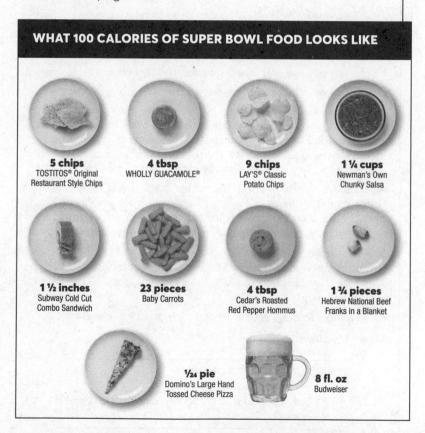

WHAT 100 CALORIES OF SUPER BOWL FOOD LOOKS LIKE

5 chips
TOSTITOS® Original
Restaurant Style Chips

4 tbsp
WHOLLY GUACAMOLE®

9 chips
LAY'S® Classic
Potato Chips

1 ¼ cups
Newman's Own
Chunky Salsa

1 ½ inches
Subway Cold Cut
Combo Sandwich

23 pieces
Baby Carrots

4 tbsp
Cedar's Roasted
Red Pepper Hommus

1 ¾ pieces
Hebrew National Beef
Franks in a Blanket

¹⁄₂₄ pie
Domino's Large Hand
Tossed Cheese Pizza

8 fl. oz
Budweiser

Buffalo Chicken Skewers with Blue-Cheese Dip

12 6- to 8-inch bamboo skewers

3 8-oz boneless, skinless chicken breasts

1 cup Louisiana-style hot sauce

¼ cup white vinegar

¼ tsp cayenne pepper

1 clove garlic, chopped

2 tsp Worcestershire sauce

2 tsp cornstarch

Blue Cheese Dip *(see step 4 below)*

1. Soak skewers in water for 60 minutes, then preheat oven to broil.

2. Cut chicken into 12 lengthwise strips; thread each strip on a skewer.

3. In a small saucepan, combine hot sauce, vinegar, cayenne pepper, garlic, and Worcestershire sauce. In a small bowl, mix cornstarch with 2 teaspoons water. Bring sauce ingredients to a boil over medium heat; add cornstarch mixture and continue cooking until sauce is slightly thickened. Remove from heat; set aside.

4. Make the blue-cheese dip in another bowl: Blend 1 cup nonfat Greek yogurt, 2 cloves garlic, chopped; 2 scallions, chopped; ¼ cup blue cheese, crumbled; and ¼ teaspoon ground black pepper. Garnish with a sprinkle of cayenne pepper, if desired; set aside.

5. Place skewers on broiler pan. Broil 8 to 10 minutes, until chicken is cooked through. While chicken is still hot, generously coat each skewer in the hot-sauce mixture. Pour remaining sauce into a small bowl for dipping.

6. Serve immediately with the hot sauce and blue-cheese dip.

Makes 12 skewers

NUTRITION AT A GLANCE
Per skewer, with dip:
Calories 115, Fat 3 g, Protein 18 g, Fiber 0 g,
Sodium 790 mg

Slow-Cooker Turkey Chili

1 tsp olive oil

1 lb ground turkey

1 large onion, chopped

1 clove garlic, minced

2 red bell peppers, chopped

2 cups frozen corn

1 (28-oz) can no-salt-added diced tomatoes

1 (15-oz) can low-sodium black beans, drained and rinsed

2 tbsp tomato paste

2 tbsp chili powder

1 tsp cumin

½ tsp cayenne pepper

½ tsp salt

⅛ tsp cinnamon

¼ cup fat-free sour cream

½ cup shredded cheddar cheese

1 bunch chives, snipped

1. In large skillet, heat oil and cook turkey, onion, and garlic over medium-high heat, stirring until turkey crumbles and is no longer pink; drain.

2. Spoon mixture into a 5-quart slow cooker; stir in peppers, corn, tomatoes, beans, tomato paste, chili powder, cumin, cayenne, salt, and cinnamon until well blended.

3. Cook on high for 4 to 5 hours or on low for 6 to 8 hours. Serve with sour cream, cheese, and chives.

Makes 6 servings

> **NUTRITION AT A GLANCE**
> Calories 300, Fat 6 g, Protein 29 g, Fiber 9 g, Sodium 440 mg

SPRING
How to make the most of these salad days

Spring is prime time for many vegetables including kale, cabbage and bok choy. Leafy greens like these are tops in nutrition. And now the produce section has more types of greens than ever, so it's easy to vary your intake. These five strategies will help you get the most benefit from springtime's salad days.

1. Blend your greens. Each type has unique nutrients, flavors, and textures. Romaine lettuce, for instance, adds crunch and is packed with vision-protecting vitamin A. Arugula imparts a spicy kick along with a dose of cancer-fighting isothiocyanate.

2. Not organic? Don't panic. Organic is best for lowering pesticide exposure and supporting a sustainable agriculture system. But your primary goal is to eat a lot of produce every day. Greens including kale, lettuce, and spinach were generally low in pesticides when Consumer Reports' scientists analyzed 12 years of Department of Agriculture data in 2015.

3. Get creative. For example, add natural sweetness to a kale salad with apples with our Kale Waldorf Salad on page 200. And topping a salad with chicken, beans, eggs, canned tuna or salmon, nuts, seeds, and whole grains can turn a simple salad into a satisfying meal.

4. Add fresh herbs. They're flavorful — so you may use less dressing — and healthy. Parsley and chives were in the top 20 of the CDC's produce ranking, but any herb works. Try our Lighter Vegetable Lasagna: it has a ¼ cup of parsley tucked into it. (Page 201)

5. Toss in some healthy fat. It helps us absorb the nutrients from greens and other veggies, a study from Purdue University found. If you use a good source of monounsaturated fat, you don't need much — just 3 grams. That's ¾ teaspoon of olive oil, ⅛ of an avocado, or 5 almonds. You can add more for flavor or satiety, but know that along with fat comes calories.

WHAT 100 CALORIES OF EASTER CANDY LOOKS LIKE

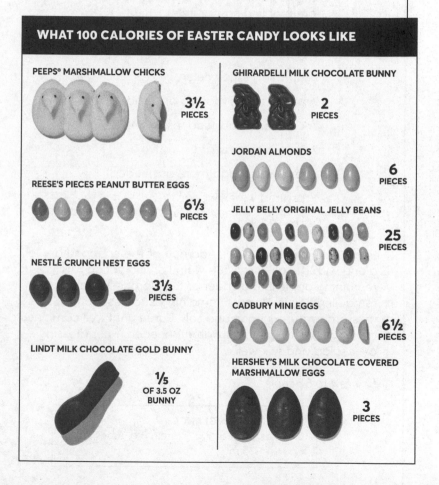

PEEPS® MARSHMALLOW CHICKS
3½ PIECES

REESE'S PIECES PEANUT BUTTER EGGS
6⅓ PIECES

NESTLÉ CRUNCH NEST EGGS
3⅓ PIECES

LINDT MILK CHOCOLATE GOLD BUNNY
⅕ OF 3.5 OZ BUNNY

GHIRARDELLI MILK CHOCOLATE BUNNY
2 PIECES

JORDAN ALMONDS
6 PIECES

JELLY BELLY ORIGINAL JELLY BEANS
25 PIECES

CADBURY MINI EGGS
6½ PIECES

HERSHEY'S MILK CHOCOLATE COVERED MARSHMALLOW EGGS
3 PIECES

Kale Waldorf Salad

4 cups packed finely chopped raw kale (preferably dinosaur kale)

1 large red apple (such as Fuji or Honeycrisp), chopped

1 cup thinly sliced celery

½ cup walnuts, toasted and chopped

¼ cup plus 2 tablespoons raisins

2 tbsp Dijon mustard

2 tbsp water (add more as needed)

1 tbsp red wine vinegar

⅛ tsp sea salt

Place kale in a large bowl. Add half of the chopped apple along with the celery, ¼ cup walnuts, and ¼ cup raisins. Put remaining apple in a blender or food processor along with remaining ¼ cup walnuts, remaining 2 tablespoons raisins, mustard, water, vinegar, and salt. Purée until well combined and slightly thick, adding water if needed. Pour dressing over salad and mix well.

Serves 4 to 6 people

NUTRITION AT A GLANCE
Calories 140, Fat 7 g, Protein 3 g, Fiber 3 g,
Sodium 135 mg

Lighter Vegetable Lasagna

1 tbsp olive oil

1 medium onion, chopped

1 small red bell pepper, chopped

8 oz baby bella mushrooms, chopped

1 small zucchini, chopped

2 cloves of garlic, minced

1 jar (25-oz) tomato basil sauce

1 container (16-oz) low-fat small-curd cottage cheese

1 egg white

¼ cup grated Parmesan cheese

¼ cup parsley leaves

8 oz part-skim mozzarella cheese, cut into cubes

¼ tsp each salt and pepper

9 oven-ready lasagna noodles

1. Heat oven to 400°F.

2. Heat oil in a large skillet over medium-high heat. Add onion, pepper, mushrooms, and zucchini. Cook about 10 minutes, stirring frequently until vegetables are soft and liquid has evaporated. Add garlic. Cook 1 minute, stirring. Add sauce and simmer 20 minutes, partially covered.

3. Meanwhile, place cottage cheese, egg white, Parmesan cheese, and parsley leaves in container of food processor. Process until smooth. Transfer into bowl and stir in mozzarella, salt, and pepper.

4. Spread ¼ of the vegetable sauce mixture into a 9x13-inch baking dish; spread to cover. Top with 3 noodles, ½ of the cheese mixture, and another ¼ of the sauce. Repeat process one more time and top with remaining sauce. Spray aluminum foil with cooking spray and cover lasagna.

5. Bake covered 25 to 30 minutes or until bubbling. Uncover and bake 5 to 10 minutes more. Let sit 10 minutes before serving.

Makes about 9 servings

NUTRITION AT A GLANCE
Calories 250, Fat 8 g, Protein 17 g, Fiber 3 g, Sodium 620 mg

---

SUMMER

How to make the most of every picnic and barbecue bash

Summertime and the cooking can be quick and easy. Fresh-from-the-farm fruits and vegetables are so good this time of year that you don't need to do much to them. Sure, there are some tricky times, even in this most easy-going season — but with a few smart tweaks, you won't have to trade in your burger for grilled veggies. You can cook up a more nutritious — but just as delicious — burger with these 5 steps:

Eat *THIS*

WATERMELON

Watermelon is one of the few foods that are packed with lycopene, a phytonutrient that appears to protect against some cancers, and may also help protect against heart disease. Plus watermelon supplies a bounty of vitamins and minerals such as B vitamins, potassium, vitamin A, and vitamin C — all for the very low cost of just 46 calories per cup. Tomatoes, pink and red grapefruit, and guava are among the other lycopene-rich foods. For a healthy, delicious treat, try the Tomato Watermelon Salad on page 206.

1. *Upgrade your bun* — and then pare it down. Starting with a 100% whole-grain, seeded burger bun adds filling fiber and other nutrients to your meal. But do keep in mind that even better-for-you carb choices can still be oversized. A 3-oz whole-wheat roll from *Great Harvest Bread Co.*, for instance, can run you 250 calories and 37 grams of carbs.

For a carb- and calorie-friendlier bun, try this: Slice rolls crosswise into three pieces rather than two. Save the middle piece for toast the next morning.

2. *Blend your beef.* You've probably gotten the memo that lean meat is your best bet, nutrition-wise. But lean beef leads to dry burgers. To add moisture to your burger, replace a third of the ground beef with roughly chopped, cooked (roasted, grilled, or broiled) mushrooms. This creates a burger that is 30 percent bigger but is still lower in calories than a traditional burger would be — and also adds an extra helping of produce.

3. Add some herbs. Grilling beef, poultry, pork, or fish results in the formation of harmful compounds that can cause changes in DNA that might increase the risk of cancer according to the National Cancer Institute.

There are several ways to cut back on the compounds, say researchers. For example, adding rosemary extract to beef patties before cooking cuts the formation of one type of compound by more than 90 percent according to one study from Kansas State University. Other research has found thyme, black pepper, ginger, and garlic also inhibit their formation. Other strategies: Keep flame low to avoid contact with the meat, and flip your burgers frequently as they cook to prevent charring.

4. Cook it completely. Foodborne illness peaks in the summer according to the USDA; using caution when you barbecue can help cut your chances of getting sick. The safest strategy is to use a meat thermometer to make sure your burgers are cooked to at least 160°F, the minimum internal temperature to destroy harmful bacteria. "If you don't have one, cook the burger until there's no pink and the juices run clear," says James E. Rogers, Ph.D., the director of food safety research and testing at Consumer Reports. "But be aware that these aren't always reliable indicators of doneness." And be sure to use a fresh plate for cooked burgers — the tray you brought the raw patties out on could be contaminated.

5. *Pile on plant power.* Often, toppings are where a burger's nutrition really goes off the rails — bacon-chili-cheeseburger, anyone? Instead, use the space between your burger and bun to add in a full serving of produce. For example, for more flavor and nutrients, upgrade the standard limp iceberg lettuce and a pale tomato piece for microgreens and a thick slice of heirloom tomato.

WHAT 100 CALORIES OF PICNIC FOOD LOOKS LIKE

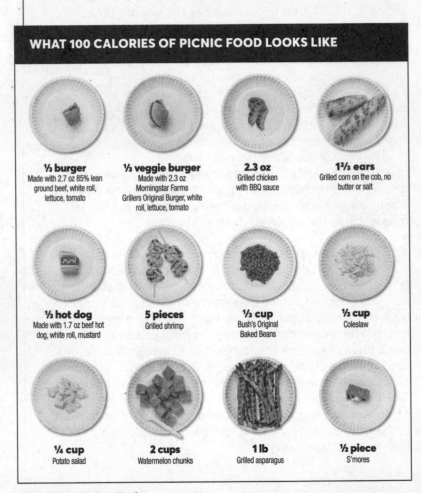

½ burger
Made with 2.7 oz 85% lean ground beef, white roll, lettuce, tomato

⅓ veggie burger
Made with 2.3 oz Morningstar Farms Grillers Original Burger, white roll, lettuce, tomato

2.3 oz
Grilled chicken with BBQ sauce

1⅔ ears
Grilled corn on the cob, no butter or salt

½ hot dog
Made with 1.7 oz beef hot dog, white roll, mustard

5 pieces
Grilled shrimp

⅓ cup
Bush's Original Baked Beans

½ cup
Coleslaw

¼ cup
Potato salad

2 cups
Watermelon chunks

1 lb
Grilled asparagus

½ piece
S'mores

CAN ICE CREAM BE HEALTHY?

More "healthy" frozen treats are appearing in the supermarket freezer case. For people watching their cholesterol, blood sugar, or weight, these products can take some of the cons out of having a cone — if you choose carefully.

LIGHT ICE CREAM

It has either at least 50-percent-less fat or 33-percent-fewer calories than a company's regular brand (or a competitor's).

PROS: It offers a significant savings in calories and fat.

CONS: While lower in fat and calories, these products usually have about the same amount of sugars as regular versions.

TREATS WITH "BENEFITS"

These are lower-sugar light ice creams or frozen desserts made with water and whey protein. They carry claims about low calories or sugars or high protein or fiber.

PROS: In vanilla flavors of some brands, you get 35 to 60 calories, 0 to 2 grams of fat, and 3 to 5 grams of sugars per half cup.

CONS: Some have no more protein than regular ice cream. And as for fiber, it's added in the form of chicory root, guar fiber, or "prebiotic" fiber. The health benefits of these types of fiber may not have the same health benefits as fiber found naturally in food.

VEGAN "ICE CREAMS"

These frozen desserts are made from almond, coconut, soy, or other plant milks, and sometimes pea protein.

PROS: They are a boon for vegans, who eat no animal products. And being dairy-free makes the desserts a benefit to people who suffer from lactose intolerance.

CONS: The ones made with coconut have saturated fat levels similar to ice cream.

Tomato Watermelon Salad

1 large seedless watermelon, cut into 1-inch cubes

4 tomatoes, cut into 1-inch dice

12 mint leaves, sliced thinly

1 large sweet onion, thinly sliced

1 cup crumbled feta cheese

¼ tbsp olive oil

2 tbsp white balsamic vinegar

Pinch coarse salt, or to taste

Pinch ground black pepper, or to taste

1. Gently mix watermelon, tomatoes, mint, onion, and feta cheese in a large bowl.

2. Whisk olive oil, vinegar, salt, and pepper together in small bowl; drizzle over salad and gently toss to coat.

Makes 12 servings

NUTRITION AT A GLANCE
Calories 314, Fat 8.5 g, Protein 6.9 g,
Fiber 3.8 g, Sodium 151 mg

Recipe from *Allrecipes*

FALL
25 tips to get you through the season's hurdles

The stretch of time from Thanksgiving through the end of the year, though joyful, can be demanding — physically, emotionally, gastronomically, and it can take a toll on your health.

The stress that often accompanies the holiday season can interfere with your immune system, making you more vulnerable to colds and possibly reducing the amount of protection you get from a flu vaccine. And even holiday happiness can have its consequences if it leads you to enjoy yourself too much at the dinner table. Many Americans consume around 4,500 calories at an average Thanksgiving feast of turkey, gravy, side dishes, and dessert. That's double the amount of calories most people should eat in a day.

Thankfully, there are ways to lighten the emotional and physical weight of the holidays. Here are 25 tips to help you navigate the season in good health.

IN THE KITCHEN

1. *Cooking for a small crowd?* Serve a turkey breast (no skin), which has about 60 fewer calories per 3.5-ounce portion than dark meat. It also cooks in less time than a whole bird.

2. *Keep chestnuts on hand.* They have less fat and about half the calories of regular nuts. Use them in stuffing and salads or as snacks.

3. *Season strategically.* Flavors like cinnamon, cloves, ginger, and nutmeg capture the essence of the season without adding many calories. Replace salt with savory basil, garlic, rosemary, sage, tarragon, thyme, or turmeric in casseroles, stuffings, and dressings.

HOW MANY CALORIES ARE IN YOUR THANKSGIVING DINNER?

APPETIZERS

147 cal.
3 PIGS IN A
BLANKET

70 cal.
1 PASTRY
BITE

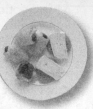

80 cal.
2 CRACKERS

95 cal.
1 OZ
BRIE CHEESE

MAIN MEAL

187 cal.
4 OZ
CANDIED
SWEET
POTATO

227 cal.
1/2 CUP
GREEN BEAN
CASSEROLE

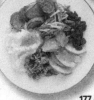

125 cal.
5 FL OZ
WINE

198 cal.
3" X 3" SQUARE
CORNBREAD

237 cal.
1 CUP MASHED
POTATOES

195 cal.
½ CUP STUFFING

25 cal.
¼ CUP GRAVY

102 cal.
1/4 CUP
CRANBERRY SAUCE

177 cal.
3½ OZ OF WHITE MEAT
TURKEY WITH SKIN

DESSERT

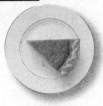

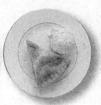

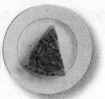

316 cal.
1 SLICE PUMPKIN PIE

411 cal.
1 SLICE APPLE PIE

137 cal.
½ CUP ICE CREAM

500 cal.
1 SLICE PECAN PIE

4. Make a healthier mash. Reduced-fat or no-fat versions of Greek yogurt taste rich and creamy and can be folded into mashed potatoes in place of butter or sour cream.

5. Bake with puréed fruit. It can replace up to 25 percent of the butter or oil in baking, cutting down on fat and calories. For instance, try plums in a chocolate cake, or applesauce in muffins or brownies. And, for a clever way to get more veggies without really trying, see our Surprise Brownie recipe on page 175.

6. Prepare poultry safely. Buy a fresh bird one or two days before you plan to cook it. Allow a frozen turkey to thaw 24 hours in the refrigerator for every 4 to 5 pounds. Don't rinse the bird: it can cause bacteria from the bird to splatter all over.

Cook turkey to a minimum internal temperature of 165°F. Check the temperature in three areas: breast, thickest part of thigh, and wing.

AT THE TABLE

7. For appetizers, think fresh. Boiled shrimp with lemon or cocktail sauce is a smarter pick than fried hors d'oeuvres. Other healthful starters include stuffed mushrooms, sliced low-fat cheese, and raw veggies with hummus.

8. Don't fast before the feast. It will probably lead to overeating. Instead, grab some small, low-calorie snacks beforehand.

9. Be mindful of how much you are eating. Consider this: A study of heart-attack patients suggested that an unusually large meal — packed with carbohydrates, fat, and salt — quadrupled the chance of having a heart attack within the next two hours.

10. *Just say no.* Peer pressure never gets easier to handle. But if you're being urged by a host to keep eating when you're full, this polite but firm statement should be able to do the trick: "No thank you, I've had enough. Everything was delicious." Or try this trick:

> **Research has found that hosts remember which guests took second (or even third) helpings, but not the amount of food they took — or ate. So you can flatter them without overeating. Take a second helping... really. Just keep both helpings small.**

11. *Relearn buffet eating.* Scan the table and make your choices before you load up a plate. You wouldn't order one of everything on a menu, so you might not want to take one of everything at a buffet.

12. *Skip the whip.* Whipped cream can add 100 calories or more when used as a drink or dessert topper. Try going without or opt for a nonfat version.

13. *Eat slowly.* For most people, incidents of heartburn are episodic and result from eating too much too fast.

14. *Sip tea.* You can cut calories by choosing tea over soda throughout the holidays. Try drinking it without sugar or milk. And tea has health benefits too. (See page 82.)

AT THE PARTY
15. *Choose spirits that are lighter colored.* Dark liquors like whiskey are more apt to cause hangovers than colorless or lighter drinks because they have more congeners, which are substances produced during fermentation that can make you feel ill.

16. Make a spritzer. Mix half red or white wine and half seltzer in a wine glass, add a slice of lime, and you have a festive drink for half the calories and alcohol content.

17. Outsmart a hangover. Don't waste your money on hangover cures that claim they'll sop up the toxic byproducts of alcohol. There's very little evidence that they will prevent or chase away a hangover. Remember, the only sure way to prevent a hangover is not to overdo it or to not drink at all. (See Go Ahead and Wine, page 79.)

FOR YOUR BODY AND SPIRIT
18. Rock 'n' clean. Nobody ever said cleaning can't be fun. OK, maybe they did, but cleaning is a great way to burn calories while whittling down your to-do list. Some fast-paced holiday tunes should get you going.

19. Forgive. Disagreements within families are normal. Don't let them ruin your holidays or health. A positive attitude can help mend and preserve relationships and also improve your heart rate and blood pressure.

20. Don't count on losing it later. If you need motivation not to put on weight over the holidays, consider this: Research shows that the extra pounds people gain during the season aren't lost during the remainder of the year.

ON YOUR TO-DO LIST
21. Hydrate. Drinking plenty of water throughout the day — at least eight glasses — will keep you from eating when you're actually thirsty.

22. Re-gift. Take food baskets or high-calorie presents you receive to work or parties so that they can be shared.

23. Keep a food diary. The more honest you are about what you eat in a day, the bigger the boost in willpower.

24. Check your doctor's vacation schedule. Make any necessary backup plans if he or she is going to be away at the end of the year. One possible reason fatal heart attacks spike during the holidays is because people wait to go to the doctor or hospital after initial symptoms appear, possibly due to a lack of available care.

25. Remember: Life isn't perfect. Stay calm and enjoy your family, friends, and all the festivities...

...and enjoy dessert! Sure, traditional Thanksgiving desserts are some of the the biggest calorie bombs of the day. If you'd like a tasty and lighter version of pumpkin pie, try Crustless Pumpkin Pie. (Recipe on page 213).

It has just 130 calories per slice vs. the 316 for typical pumpkin pie. You save 186 calories per slice. It might just be the perfect ending to your Thanksgiving meal.

Crustless Pumpkin Pie

15-oz can pumpkin puree

12-oz can fat-free evaporated milk

½ cup light brown sugar

1 egg plus 2 egg whites from large eggs

1 tsp pumpkin pie spice

1 tsp vanilla extract

4 ginger snap cookies, crushed

1. Heat oven to 350°F. Spray 9-inch glass pie pan with nonstick spray.

2. In a large bowl whisk together pumpkin, milk, sugar, eggs, pumpkin pie spice and vanilla until well blended.

3. Spoon into prepared pan. Bake 45-50 minutes or until the filling jiggles like JELL-O™ when the plate is gently moved.

4. Cool completely. Right before serving sprinkle with crushed ginger snaps.

Makes 8 servings

NUTRITION AT A GLANCE
Calories 130, Fat 1.5 g, Fiber 2 g, Protein 6 g, Sodium 80 mg

---

SHOULD I EAT THIS?
AN ANSWER TO THE QUESTION

By now, if you've read through the pages of this book, you have a good idea of what you *should* and *should not* eat.

For example, you know that you should eat Brazil nuts to power up your memory, apples to control your blood pressure, and peas to help keep your muscles strong. And you know that you should never eat any food with "partially hydrogenated oils" on the label.

And of course, when it comes to deciding whether you should or should not eat something, there are variables. Your age, weight, height, sex, and overall health are all factors. But generally speaking, for healthy people, there is one simple rule that can guide you:

Don't overeat. If you are full, the answer to the question, *Should I Eat This?* is *no*.

You may be tempted to break this rule. But science shows that overeating is not in your best interest. Any food eaten beyond what your body needs for energy, growth, regeneration, and healing brings you no physiological benefit. Overindulgence, even of what we think of as "healthy" foods, can cause weight gain, inflammation, and imbalances in the body.

If you keep this rule in mind, little by little it can become a part of your life. And it will work for you to help boost your memory, protect your heart, prevent disease, maintain a healthy weight and stay strong.

Then, along with the information in this book, you will know the answer to the question: *Should I Eat This?*

INDEX